PRIMER OF
GASTROINTESTINAL
FIBEROPTIC ENDOSCOPY

CHOICHI SUGAWA, M.D.

Associate Professor of Surgery
Wayne State University School of Medicine
Chief, Surgical Endoscopy Unit
Detroit Receiving Hospital
Detroit, Michigan

BERNARD M. SCHUMAN, M.D.

Clinical Associate Professor of Internal Medicine
University of Michigan Medical School
Ann Arbor, Michigan
Division Head, Gastroenterology
Henry Ford Hospital
Detroit, Michigan

PRIMER OF GASTROINTESTINAL FIBEROPTIC ENDOSCOPY

FOREWORD BY
ALEXANDER J. WALT, M.B., Ch.B.
Chairman, Department of Surgery
Wayne State University School of Medicine
Detroit, Michigan

LITTLE, BROWN
AND COMPANY
BOSTON

TO NATSUKO AND SARAH

CONTENTS

It is an unusual ecumenical experience to watch a book designed to fill a void in the literature take shape so happily under the authorship of two individuals who come from such completely different backgrounds. With the advent of flexible fiberoptic instruments, the field of endoscopy has made tremendous strides over the past decade. Not surprisingly, physicians trained in different disciplines often have an equal interest but different perspective as they view lesions of the gastrointestinal tract. On occasion, the fences between the medical and surgical specialties in this area display an artificiality born of clinical custom. Doctor Choichi Sugawa and Doctor Bernard Schuman have sought to remove these barriers and to take the mystery out of endoscopy. In the course of this endeavor, they have produced a practical, orderly, well-organized guide for physicians from all specialties who seek to develop a basic understanding of the field.

Doctor Schuman, as head of the Division of Gastroenterology at the Henry Ford Hospital in Detroit, and Doctor Sugawa, the Chief of Surgical Endoscopy at Wayne State University, have pooled their vast experience in the design of this book. In many ways, this combined effort has been a model of synergism. Doctor Schuman, past president of the American Society for Gastrointestinal Endoscopy, has long been preeminent in this field. Doctor Sugawa, in turn, is noted for his fundamental work in the laboratory, and for his acute endoscopy in the critically ill patient. These two experts, both of whom have been deeply involved in the training of residents, have produced a book replete with practical suggestions.

Doctor Sugawa first came to the United States from Japan in 1969 as a research fellow, already a trained surgeon in the area of upper gastrointestinal surgical disease, bringing with him a gastrocamera and a thorough knowledge of endoscopy. Working in the laboratory and in the clinic in a completely integrated manner, Doctor Sugawa took ideas from one milieu to the other, recognizing the vast potential of the camera and the flexible endoscope in the study of sequential gastric responses to disease. Later Doctor Sugawa extended his interest to the pancreas as ERCP became available; he has made considerable contributions in this area too, bringing a surgical flavor to his approach.

Doctor Schuman has been a widely acknowledged pioneer in the field of endoscopy and a leader in gastroenterology for more than a decade. Active as a clinician and responsible for the training of gastroenterologists, Doctor Schuman is nationally recognized for his contributions to the acquisition of new knowledge and for his efforts to ensure that endoscopy is performed for the right reasons in the right manner. His judgment and wisdom as a practicing physician permeate the text.

This joint effort of two experts from different disciplines and different institutions serves as a model of cooperation for physicians working in the field of endoscopy. The lucidity of their book, born of their pioneering experiences and extensive clinical exposure, makes it much easier for the rest of us to gain endoscopic skills in a much less painful way, both for our patients and ourselves.

Alexander J. Walt

The majority of books and journal reviews related to the field of gastrointestinal endoscopy are addressed to the physician who is already experienced in and practicing fiberoptic endoscopy. It seemed to us that there was a need for an introductory text to accompany the student of fiberoptic endoscopy during his supervised training. Forearmed with the knowledge of available instrumentation, techniques of intubation, and the more common pathologic lesions to be encountered, the student's receptiveness to his training would be enhanced.

We also believed that it was important to describe the major techniques available to the digestive tract endoscopist in one book. It is evident now that fiberoptic endoscopy is not necessarily the prerogative of the gastroenterologist. Upper gastrointestinal endoscopy has become of interest to physicians in many branches of medicine, including internal medicine, family practice, pediatrics, general surgery, and radiology. Obviously, in a community where a trained endoscopist is not available, a physician in an appropriate specialty will seek out opportunities for short-term training in order to provide this important diagnostic service. Endoscopy cannot be learned from a book, but a book will supplement the personal instruction provided in the endoscopy suite, so that the trainee will recognize the problems and avoid the pitfalls.

Unlike the gastroenterologist, other physicians undertaking endoscopy may be concerned with only one or two techniques. The general surgeon may be interested in either upper gastrointestinal endoscopy or colonoscopy, and would consider his time better spent doing choledochoscopy rather than endoscopic retrograde cholangiopancreatography. The colon and rectal surgeon, on the other hand, will obviously concentrate his efforts on fiberoptic sigmoidoscopy and colonoscopy. In the clinical setting of internal medicine or family practice, upper gastrointestinal endoscopy may be the only procedure that would be called on frequently enough to maintain the skills of the physician. Recognizing the variety of interests, we have attempted to bring together the basic information needed to begin training in any of the digestive tract endoscopic procedures.

Our goal was not to provide an exhaustive compendium of all available information on gastrointestinal endoscopy but rather to present a concise overview of the state of the art. We recognize that there may be undue emphasis on aspects in which one or the other of us has had a special experience, but we feel that the dual authorship by both a surgeon and a gastroenterologist maintains a "check and balance"; neither author gets carried away in his specialty. Selected references have been chosen on the basis of historic importance as well as currency of thought and, although not readily accessible, foreign contributions (particularly from Japan and Germany) are cited because of the major contributions made by the authors from those countries to the field of endoscopy of the gastrointestinal tract.

Members of the American Society for Gastrointestinal Endoscopy (ASGE) have, through their work in committees of the society, provided much factual material, to which we have frequently referred. For example, we have used the data on complications of fiberoptic endoscopy obtained from surveys of the membership; the conclusions, therefore, take on greater reliability than a mere collection of individual reports. In addition, we recommend to our readers statements on specific indications for endoscopy that represent the combined effort of several experienced endoscopists of ASGE. These official publications, as well as "Guidelines on Training and Standards of Practice," can be obtained by writing the Executive Secretary, American Society for Gastrointestinal Endoscopy, P.O. Box 1565, Manchester, Massachusetts 01944.

We are indebted to medical students, residents in medicine and surgery, gastroenterology fellows, and practicing physicians who, by asking questions, provide the motivation to examine constantly what we are doing endoscopically. We acknowledge with thanks the contributions that some of our surgical and gastroenterologic colleagues have made to several of the authors' studies that are reviewed in the text. We are grateful for the secretarial assistance provided by Ms. Sherry L. Doggett, who accepted so graciously every new revision of the manuscript.

C.S.

B.M.S.

PRIMER OF
GASTROINTESTINAL
FIBEROPTIC ENDOSCOPY

CHAPTER 1

HISTORY OF GASTROINTESTINAL FIBEROPTIC ENDOSCOPY

It is unlikely that any physician who graduated from medical school after 1970 has handled other than the fiberoptic gastrointestinal endoscopes. Indeed, the young physician probably has not seen a rigid endoscope unless he or she has visited a medical museum or observed the exhibit on the development of gastrointestinal endoscopy sponsored by the American Society for Gastrointestinal Endoscopy. Those doctors who have used the semirigid or semiflexible (depending on your point of view) instruments can better appreciate the revolutionary advance in only the last 10 years that fiberoptic endoscopy represents in the diagnosis of digestive tract disease.

It was over 100 years ago that the first attempt to visualize the stomach with a rigid tube was made by Kussmaul, who believed that the contour of the upper gastrointestinal tract would straighten when a metal tube was introduced from the mouth into the stomach. Rigid esophagoscopy developed over the next 50 years, progress being primarily dependent on the design of a good light source. However, efforts to construct a successful gastroscope, although imaginative, were doomed to fail because the rigid instrument was able to survey only a small portion of the stomach, and carried a significant hazard of perforation.

In 1932, a semiflexible instrument was designed by Schindler and Wolf, and the Schindler gastroscope remained the blueprint for development of gastroscopes for the next 30 years. The semiflexible gastroscope was based on the principle that a series of convex lens can transmit light undistorted through a flexible tube if the distal tube is not bent beyond a certain angle. Thus more of the gastric surface could be examined although important blind areas still remained, and the risk of perforation was reduced particularly by the placement of a rubber obturator at the tip. When Schindler came to Chicago in the mid-1930s and demonstrated the value of semiflexible gastroscopy, many physicians from teaching centers all over the United States came to him for instruction in the tecnnique. Gastroscopy, however, remained a technique utilized by relatively few gastroenterologists.

In 1958, Hirschowitz, Curtiss, Peters, and Pollard published their report of a new gastroscope, the fiberscope. This revolutionary instrument had its genesis 30 years earlier, when Baird showed that light could travel the entire length of a curved glass tube. Baird's discovery led to the production by Hopkins and Caponni in 1954 of the clad glass fiber which, through the phenomenon of total internal reflection, allowed light to travel from one end to another regardless of how the fiberglass was coiled.

The flexible fiberoptic gastroscope engineered by Curtiss was first clinically employed by Dr. Basil Hirschowitz in early 1957 at the University Hospital in Ann Arbor, Michigan. It was a side-viewing instrument useful primarily for examination of the stomach. Ultimately it became obvious that a forward-viewing instrument would be necessary if the esophagus were to be examined. The American Cystoscope Makers, Inc. (ACMI), which initiated the commercial manufacture of fiberoptic instruments, produced a fiberoptic esophagoscope with the clinical guidance of Lo Presti. Thereafter it was demonstrated by Belber and others that it was possible to intubate the duodenum and to visualize the duodenal bulb with a gastroscope. The development of fiberoptic instruments for examination of the upper gastrointestinal tract then proceeded by leaps and bounds in the United States, in Japan, and in Europe with the production of a fiberoptic panendoscope for examination of the esophagus, stomach, and duodenum by 1970.

The development of fiberoptic colonoscopy proceeded along similar lines. In 1961, Overholt initiated the use of a fiberoptic sigmoidoscope, and later described techniques for successful examination of the rectum and sigmoid colon. Instrument design was improved by the engineers at ACMI and at the Olympus Corporation, with the result that by the early 1970s it was possible to examine the entire colon. Intubation techniques were refined by Shinya who reported his experience with a large number of patients. Thereafter Shinya and Wolff devised the technique of polypectomy using a snare and electrocoagulation. By 1975, total colonoscopy with snare polypectomy was a commonplace procedure throughout the world.

At the World Congress of Gastroenterology in 1970, Oi presented his work on endoscopic retrograde cholangiopancreatography (ERCP). Employing a specially designed side-viewing duodenoscope, he was able to intubate the orifice of the major papilla of the duodenum successfully in a high percentage of patients. Although considerable effort and patience were required to learn this technique, it was soon being performed in several centers in Japan. Vennes introduced ERCP in the United States and trained many American doctors, who in turn taught the method to colleagues and trainees in residency programs. The procedure became available to patients in practically every major hospital in the country.

Recent developments with ERCP have brought about a method of introduction of a "daughter" scope into the common bile duct and pancreatic duct for direct endoscopic visualization. This technique *is* still in its infancy; to what extent it will prove valuable in diagnosis or management of disease is as yet undetermined.

As an outgrowth of ERCP, Kawai and Soma in Japan and Demling and Classen in Germany designed a papillotome that can be introduced through the biopsy channel of the duodenoscope, so that an incision of the major papilla with electrocoagulation can be performed. Endoscopic papillotomy has become a successful method of treatment for retained common bile duct stones, and has been used in many patients in Europe, and to a lesser extent in the United States.

The growth and development of gastrointestinal endoscopy from 1957 to the present has been nothing less than phenomenal. Fiberoptic technology transformed gastroscopy from an infrequently requested and often mistrusted, limited procedure into a safe, highly acceptable endoscopic method, surpassing radiologic examination of the upper gastrointestinal tract in diagnostic accuracy. Moreover, therapeutic adaptations add a new dimension to panendoscopy of the digestive tract. If innovations of the 1980s in gastrointestinal endoscopy can match only half the innovations of the 1970s, it will still be an exciting time.

SELECTED READINGS

Classen, M., and Demling, L.   Endoskopische Sphincteromie der Papilla Vateri. *Dtsch. Med. Wochenschr.* 99:496, 1974.

Gordon, M.E., and Kirsner, J.B.   Rudolf Schindler, pioneer endoscopist: Glimpses of the man and his work. *Gastroenterology* 77:354, 1979.

Hirschowitz, B.I.   A personal history of the fiberscope. *Gastroenterology* 76:864, 1979.

Hirschowitz, B.I., et al.   Demonstration of a new gastroscope, the fiberscope. *Gastroenterology* 35:50, 1958.

Kasugai, T., et al.   Endoscopic pancreatocholangiography. I. The normal endoscopic pancreatocholangiogram. II. The pathological endoscopic pancreatocholangiogram. *Gastroenterology* 63:217, 1972.

Kawai, K., et al.   Endoscopic sphincterotomy of the ampulla of Vater. *Gastrointest. Endosc.* 20:148, 1974.

Overholt, F.   Clinical experience with the fibersigmoidoscope. *Gastrointest. Endosc.* 15:27, 1968.

Schindler, R.   Gastroscopy with a flexible gastroscope. *Am. J. Dig. Dis. Nutr.* 2:656, 1936.

Soma, S.   Endoscopic sphincterotomy: A new approach for extraction of residual stones. *Gastroent. Endosc. (Japan)* 16:452, 1974.

Vennes, J.A., and Silvis, S.E.   Endoscopic visualization of bile and pancreatic ducts. *Gastrointest. Endosc.* 18:149, 1972.

Wolff, W.I., and Shinya, A.   A new approach to the management of colonic polyps. *Adv. Surg.* 7:45, 1973.

CHAPTER 2

GENERAL PRINCIPLES AND INSTRUMENTATION

THE PRINCIPLE OF LIGHT AND IMAGE TRANSMISSION THROUGH GLASS FIBERS

Fiberoptics is the unique method of conveying an image through a curve in fine long glass fibers (see Fig. 2-1). Transmission of light through flexible glass fiber bundles was demonstrated by Baird in 1928. No practical use of this important discovery was made, since the quality of the fiberglass prevented transmission of sufficient light for good visualization. The principle was established, however, that when light enters the end face of a glass fiber, it is trapped and conducted by numerous reflections in the walls of the fiber through the other end face of the fiber (see Fig. 2-2). This physical property of light transmission, the phenomenon of total internal reflection, is based on the wave theory of light first proposed by Huygens in the seventeenth century to explain refraction and reflection of light.

The most obvious demonstration of the principle of refraction or bending of light involves a beam of light traveling in air that strikes a water interface at an oblique angle. Because the velocity of light is less in water than in air, the light is refracted. Thus light traveling from air to water would have a high refractive index, and light traveling from water to air would have a low refractive index. In a medium with a low refractive index, when the light strikes the interface at a particular critical angle of incidence (instead of being refracted), the light beam is, in fact, reflected off the interface and total internal reflection occurs.

In the mid–1950s, Curtiss attempted to reduce the loss of light from fiberglass by making glass of a high refractive index. It had been previously demonstrated that a lacquer coating of the glass fiber would prevent light loss, because the lacquer had a lower refractive index than the glass. The lacquer coating was not uniform, however, and light leaks occurred, reducing the transmission of light when the glass fibers were put into a bundle. Curtiss found that a fiber of high refractive index could be coated with glass of a lower refractive index. His fiber, therefore, consisted of a core fiber 10 μ thick, clad with glass 1 μ in thickness. Glass fibers less than 10 μ in diameter will not trap light with a wavelength measuring 0.4 to 0.7 μ. Thus the present fiber bundles produce the best possible resolution.

Fiberglass is bundled and used either for illumination or for the transmission of images. A fiber bundle made to illuminate need not have its component glass fibers arranged in any particular order. This

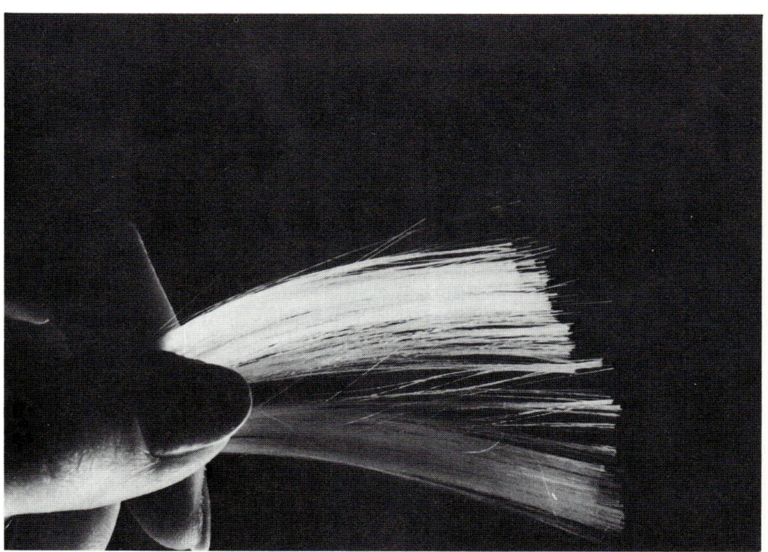

Figure 2-1.   A bundle of glass fibers.

kind of bundle is called an incoherent bundle, and a glass fiber with a diameter of 25 μ will suffice for this purpose. An illuminating system for an endoscope consists of a light source that projects light through lenses onto the face of an incoherent flexible fiber bundle, which is then brought in contact with a similar incoherent bundle in the endoscope.

A bundle arranged so that individual glass fibers are in the same position at the distal end of the bundle as at the proximal end of the bundle is called a coherent bundle (see Fig. 2-3). Although a clad glass fiber gives almost perfect total reflection, light can be lost because of other design features. Thus, Hopkins estimated that 30 percent of the lamp light can be lost by reflections at the air glass surfaces. Since only the core glass of each fiber transmits light, light falling on the cladding or on the cement binding bundles will be lost. Loss of light at the coupling of the illuminating bundle (from the light source) and the coupling of the endoscope has been avoided by use of an integral incoherent fiber bundle. There are, however, light losses at the two end faces of the coherent bundle.

In addition to the adequacy of light transmission, Hopkins points out that the type of objective arrangement is important. A telecentric objective is required in order that the pencil of light emerging from the proximal end of the coherent bundle is not narrowed at its exit.

Figure 2-2.   Total internal reflection of light within the fiber.

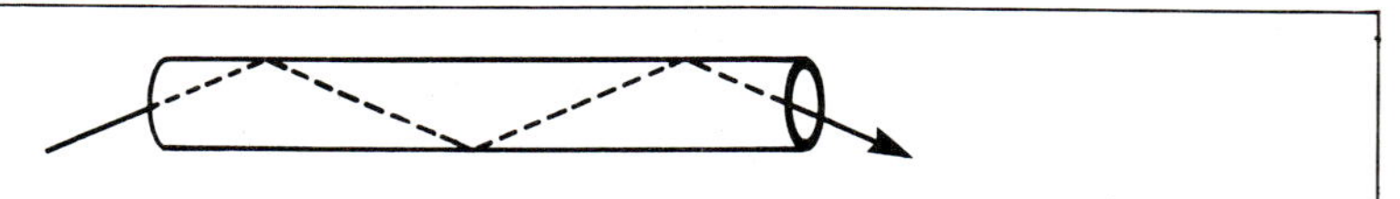

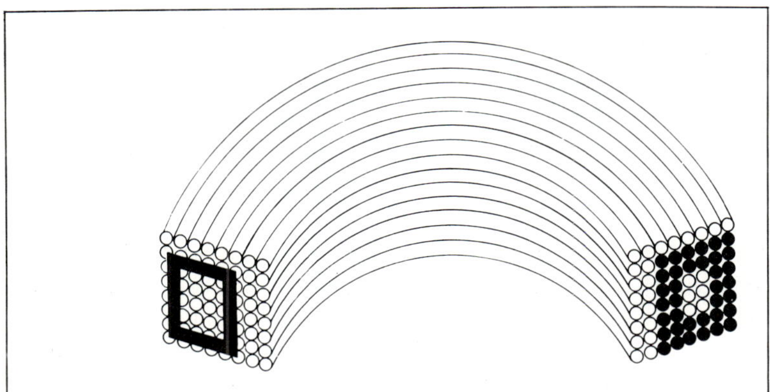

Figure 2-3.   *Point-by-point transmission via the coherent bundle.*

Ultimately, the image resolution of a fiberoptic endoscope depends on the size and spacing of the fibers in the coherent fiber bundle, and on the depth of focus of the objective lens (see Fig. 2-4). The proximal image is much like that observed on a television screen where the pic-

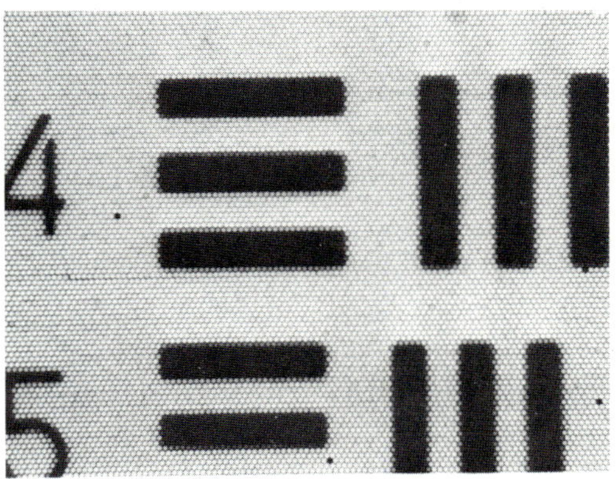

Figure 2-4.   *Mosaic of fibers forming an image.*

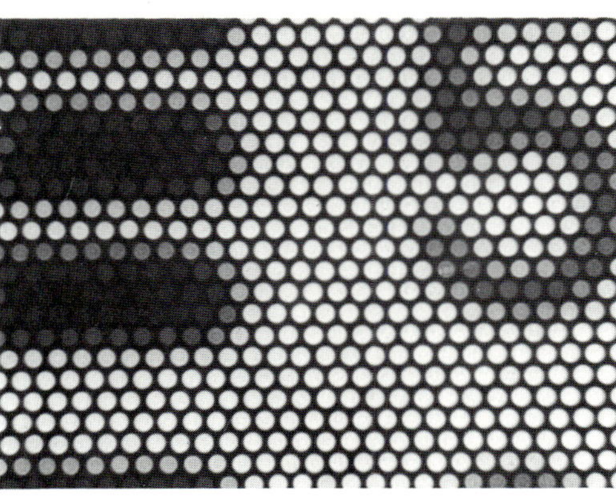

ture is the result of discrete elements; a mosaic is thus formed. The mosaic becomes more apparent in proportion to the thickness of the space between two fibers as well as to the eyepiece magnification. Since the endoscope has a fixed focus, image quality must be high to compensate for the detail that can be achieved when an exact focus can be set.

THE ENDOSCOPY ROOM AND ITS EQUIPMENT

Although gastrointestinal endoscopic procedures can be done almost anywhere from the operating room to an open area in the emergency unit, a room especially designed for fiberoptic endoscopy will allow maximum efficiency of performance. It is not necessary to tie up an operating room for this purpose. It is a rare occasion when general anesthesia is required for an endoscopy, and operating room personnel are not required for assistance that can be adequately given by anyone properly trained. Endoscopy at times must be performed in an emergency-room setting or in an intensive care unit, but the elective case is best brought to a specifically designed endoscopy room.

There should be separate rooms for upper gastrointestinal endoscopy and for colonoscopy. Because of the risk of contamination of the upper gastrointestinal endoscopes, it is unwise to perform both types of procedure in the same room. Laparoscopy, however, can be done safely in a suite set up for upper gastrointestinal endoscopy after the room has been properly cleaned.

Room for Upper Gastrointestinal Endoscopy

For upper gastrointestinal endoscopy, a room measuring 18 by 12 ft would be more than adequate (see Fig. 2-5). The examining table should be centered in the room so that there is adequate space to circulate about the table. A table that can be electronically controlled so that it moves up and down (as well as allowing the head to tilt down) is desirable if not essential. A multipurpose Ritter table can be used advantageously for upper gastrointestinal endoscopy. The room should contain adequate table top surface to ensure proximity of accessory equipment and to allow preparation of the various tissues and cytologic material obtained in the course of an examination. There should also be a desk available, so that reports can be written and records reviewed. A sink for hand-washing and a larger sink for the washing of equipment are also needed. Adequate cabinet space to hold all equipment is important. The cabinets should be tall enough that the endoscopes can be hung by the handle with the shaft of the scope hanging free (see Fig. 2-6). A bank of x-ray viewing boxes should be hung at a location where they can be readily viewed by the endos-

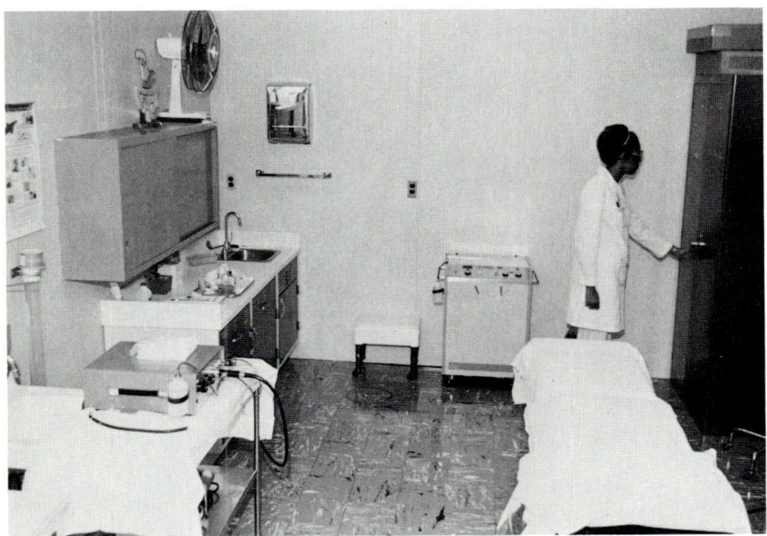

Figure 2-5. Endoscopy room for upper gastrointestinal endoscopy.

copist at the examining table if necessary. Overhead lights should be bright, and a rheostat for control of the light intensity is a convenience but not a necessity. It is a good idea to have the capability to black-out the room so that color television may be more easily viewed; at times it is helpful to be able to see the position of the endoscope light within the abdominal cavity. The door to the room should be at least 4 ft wide to allow easy access for a stretcher. Air conditioning will considerably enhance the efficiency of operation during the summer months.

Room for Colonoscopy

The room for colonoscopy should be designed in a fashion similar to that for the upper gastrointestinal endoscopy room (see Fig. 2-7). Additionally, special arrangements for cabinetry should be made so that the 180-cm colonoscope can be hung in the cabinet without its end trailing at the bottom of the cabinet. In addition to space for the light source next to the examining table, there must also be a cart to carry the electrocoagulation equipment and the accessories for the unit. Ready access to fluoroscopy is important, and although it is not necessary to perform colonoscopy on a fluoroscopic table, under certain circumstances it is advantageous to move the patient easily from an examining table to the fluoroscopic table. Providing this kind of arrangement, however, entails considerable expense not only for the fluoroscopic equipment but also for the appropriate lead lining of the room and door.

Figure 2-6.   Cabinet containing endo-scopes and accessory equipment.

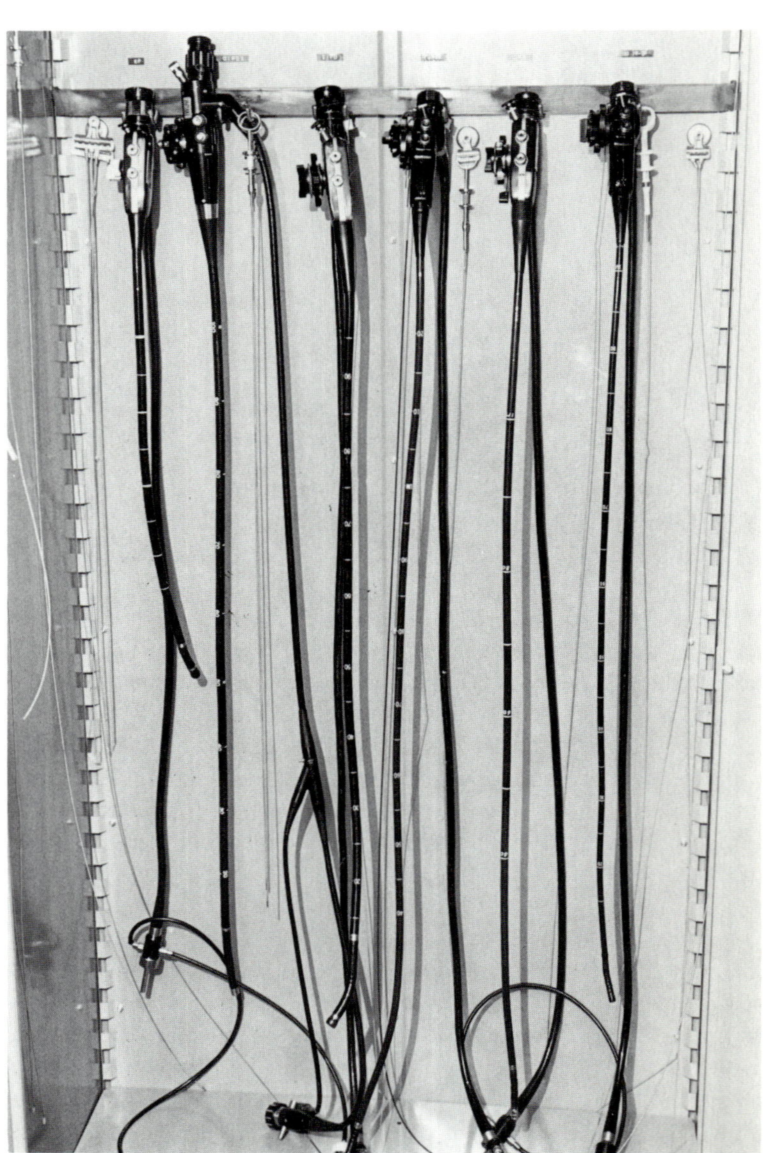

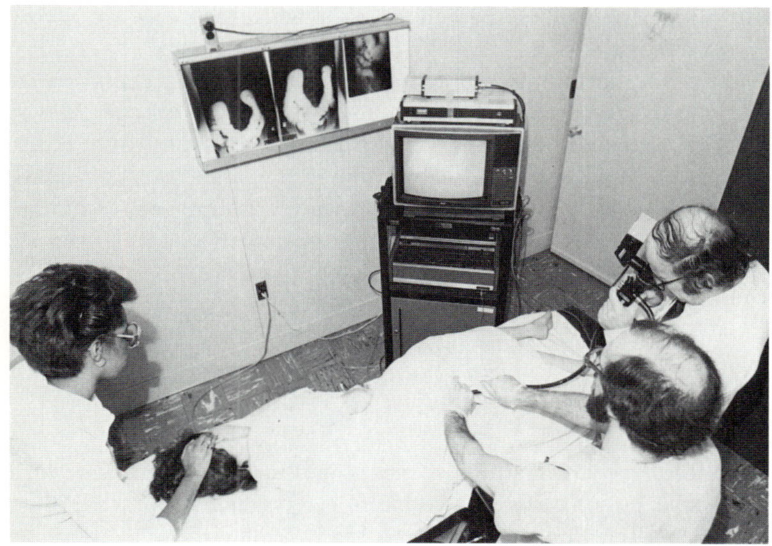

Figure 2-7.   The colonoscopy room and closed-circuit television.

Room for Endoscopic Retrograde Cholangiopancreatography (ERCP)
The expense involved in setting up an x-ray unit exclusively for endoscopic retrograde cholangiopancreatography is prohibitive for the vast majority of endoscopists. Thus ERCP is done in the x-ray department on a shared-time basis in most institutions. Not only is good fluoroscopic equipment with x-ray filming capability required, but there must also be a unit for the rapid development of film close at hand.

Personnel for the Endoscopy Room
Although a registered nurse can provide expertise and be given greater responsibility in the management of the endoscopy room and the care of equipment, a licensed practical nurse can be trained to carry out all the necessary activities of the endoscopy room, in addition to preparing the appropriate medication and giving parenteral drugs as needed. An individual merely trained as an endoscopy room technician (to carry out the functions of an assistant and maintain the instruments) is at a disadvantage when it comes to dealing with specific patient needs. Although endoscopy can be done by throwing almost anyone into the breach to act as an assistant, this method ordinarily results in an unsatisfactory examination, and may even be detrimental to the patient. Skilled assistance is essential for an informative, safe, endoscopic examination to be carried out.

The Society for Gastrointestinal Assistants has established guidelines for the training of endoscopy assistants, and provides educational opportunities that will serve to enhance the performance of the endoscopy assistant.

In teaching institutions, of course, a medical or surgical resident or fellow in gastroenterology is available first as an assistant; he gains in experience and knowledge as a working endoscopist under the supervision of his teacher. For ERCP, a radiologist in attendance is valuable and will lead to superior x-ray films, but often only an x-ray technician is available for assisting the endoscopist in obtaining the appropriate films following successful cannulation.

INSTRUMENTS, LIGHT SOURCES, AND ACCESSORY EQUIPMENT

Instruments

A complete armamentarium of endoscopes for upper gastrointestinal panendoscopy, colonoscopy, and ERCP requires the purchase of an impressive number of instruments. The mechanical components of the various types of endoscopes are essentially the same (see Fig. 2–8).

For upper gastrointestinal panendoscopy, a forward-viewing instrument is the workhorse. A side-viewing gastroduodenoscope, however, is also useful in those patients whose complete examination cannot be done with the forward-viewing instrument. A smaller caliber pediatric panendoscope is important if children are to be ex-

Figure 2-8.   An exploded view of the fiberscope.

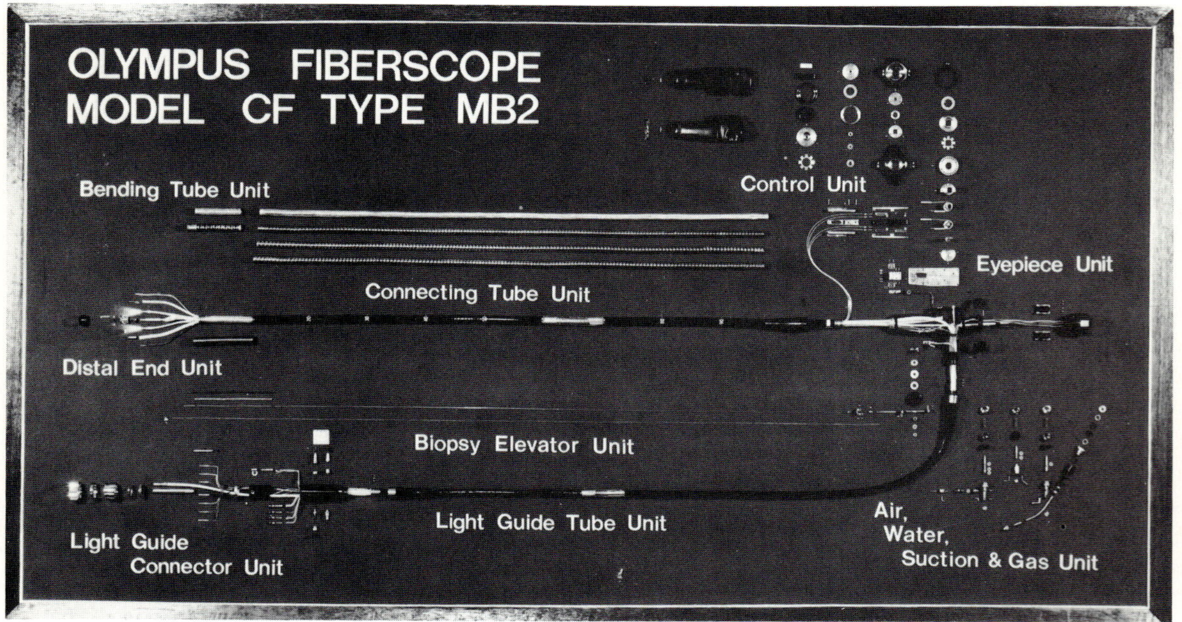

amined, and as a back-up for the standard panendoscope should it be away for repair (see Fig. 2-9). A side-viewing gastroduodenoscope is, of course, essential if ERCP is to be done.

For the colonoscopy suite, a long (180 cm) colonoscope would be the major diagnostic unit. The medium-bundle colonoscope (100–140 cm), however, is a useful back-up instrument, and in many instances may be all that is required for total or near-total colonoscopy. The 60-cm fiberoptic sigmoidoscope is also gaining in popularity as a screening instrument for patients who are at higher risk for the development of colon cancer (see Fig. 2-10A,B), but obviously the medium-bundle colonoscope will do as well.

A more detailed description of these endoscopes will be given in subsequent chapters related to specific procedures.

Light Sources

In a sense, the endoscope is only as good as the light source to which it is attached. An endoscope with a good fiberglass bundle will not pro-

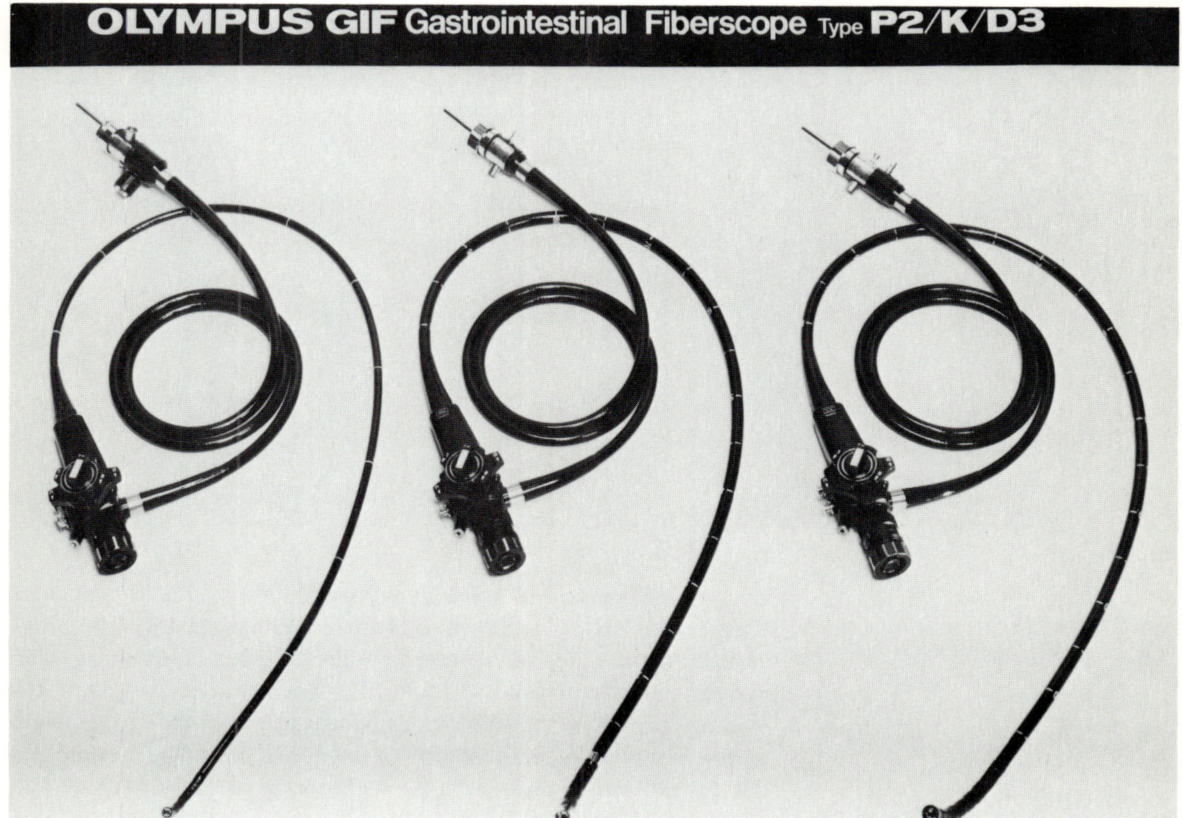

Figure 2-9.   Olympus panendoscopes for pediatric and adult patients.

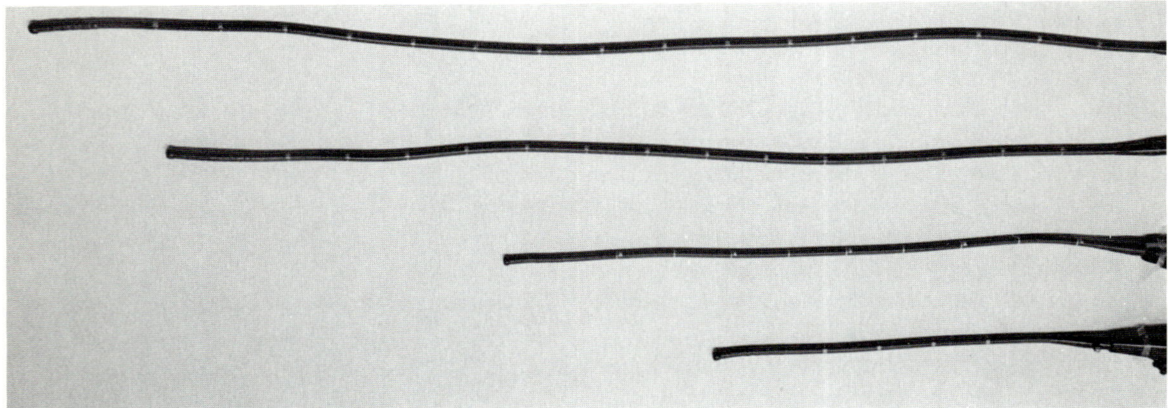

A

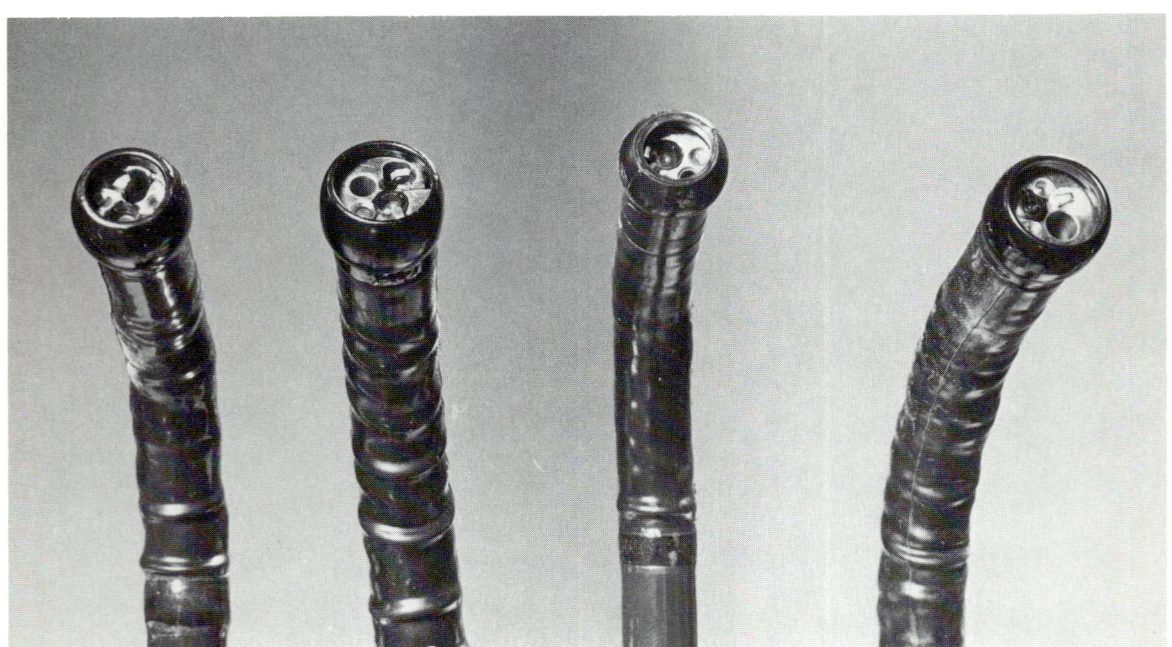

B

Figure 2-10. A. Colonoscopes of varying lengths. B. Single and double-channel colonoscopes as viewed at the tip.

duce a bright image of good quality if the light source is inadequate. The trend is toward endoscopes of smaller caliber, and therefore thinner fiberoptic light bundles that require brighter light sources than were previously available. Additionally, developments in still and cine photography as well as the more frequent use of closed-circuit television require that the light source be capable of providing an output of 300 to 500 watts. Fortunately, the engineering of lamps has kept pace

with the design changes and requirements of modern fiberoptic endoscopy.

The tungsten filament lamp has been improved by adding iodine to
the quartz cover of the filament, thus preventing the dissociation of
tungsten and increasing the amount of light available.

The halogen reflector lamp reflects most of the visible light but
filters out some of the heat-producing light, focusing the light on the
incoherent carrier fiberglass bundle (see Fig. 2-11). This type of lamp
can be found in the Olympus CLE-3 and -4U (see Fig. 2-12), in the

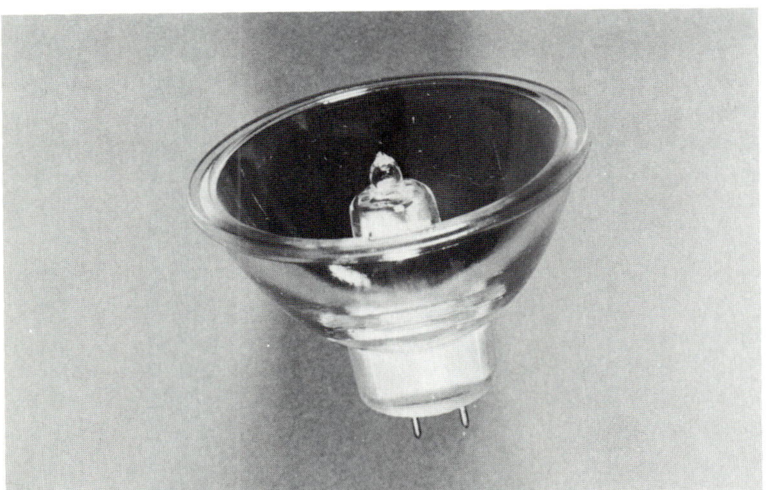

Figure 2-11.   Halogen reflector lamp.

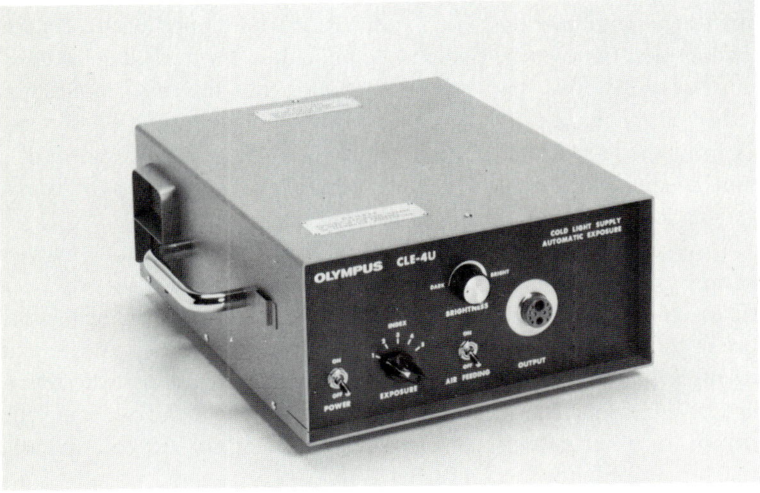

*Figure 2-12.   Olympus light source
(CLE-4U).*

ACMI 10-10, and in the Fujinon FIL-150 EF-B light sources. Xenon lamps are used in the Olympus CLX light source and the ACMI 1210 light source (see Figs. 2-13A,B), both of which give an intense ozonefree cold light with an output of over 300 watts. These light sources supply enough illumination for cine photography and for color television. Where teaching attachments are employed, there is also sufficient light so that both the endoscopist and the assistant or student can see a reasonably bright image with clarity.

Accessory Equipment

VIEWING ATTACHMENT.   A flexible fiberglass side arm is available for attachment to the eyepiece of the endoscope (see Fig. 2-14A,B). The image is split so that the endoscopist and the trainee or assistant can view the field at the same time, permitting better instruction or more coordinated manipulation. The viewing attachment should not be looked on as a toy or luxury, because it can be of considerable assistance in therapeutic maneuvers such as polypectomy. Each instrument maker has an attachment manufactured especially for its own endoscope (see Fig. 2-15), but adapters are available for interchange of teaching attachments. The adapter does lead to loss of light, however; it is best to invest in the teaching attachment at the time the endoscope is purchased.

BIOPSY FORCEPS.   Biopsy forceps are designed to pass easily through the biopsy channel of the endoscope and then be brought to bear upon the biopsy area, either by raising the tip of the endoscope or by utilizing a forceps elevator at the end of the biopsy channel. The forceps is composed of two cups of varying shape, the edges of which may be smooth or dentate (see Fig. 2-16). The size of the cup may vary from two to three millimeters. The forceps is often designed with a central bayonet that permits the tissue to be pinned down so that an accurate biopsy can be taken (see Fig. 2-17). Once the cups are brought together, the tissue is torn off and retrieved by bringing the biopsy forceps out through the channel. Excessive bleeding or perforation of a hollow viscus with a biopsy forceps is highly unlikely unless there is a coagulation disorder or unusual thinning of the wall.

A variation of the biopsy forceps is the electrocoagulating biopsy forceps (see Fig. 2-18). This "hot" biopsy forceps is insulated by a Teflon covering and attaches to an electrocoagulation snare handle, just as the polypectomy snare does. This permits biopsy excision of polyps 5 mm or less in diameter. The Teflon sheath also has the advantage of decreasing the friction in the biopsy channel and allowing the forceps to pass more readily, particularly within the colonoscope which may be looped upon itself.

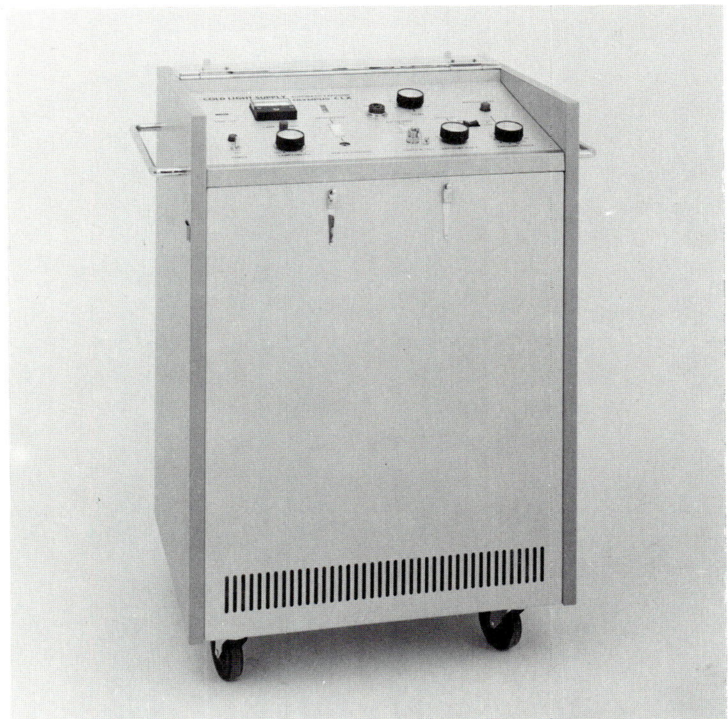

A

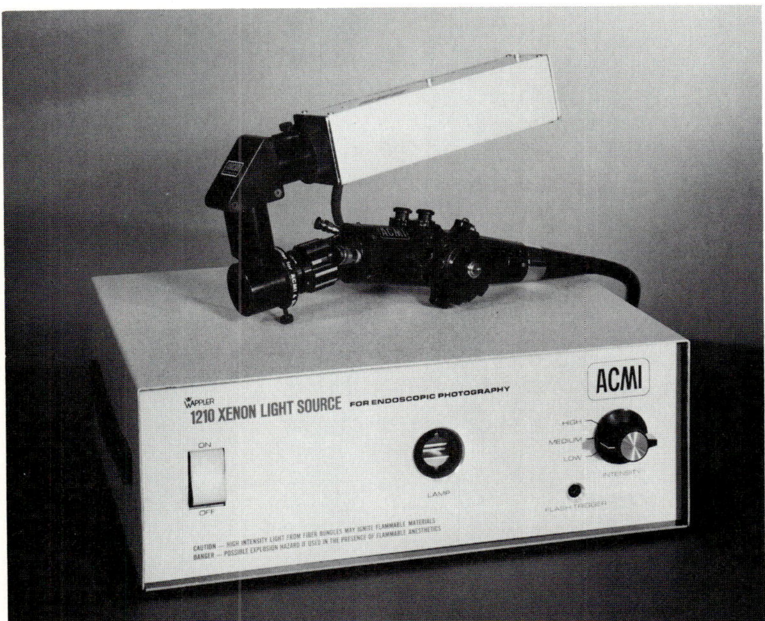

B

Figure 2-13.   A. Olympus CLX light source with xenon lamp. B. ACMI 1210 light source with xenon lamp. ACMI panendoscope is fitted with the circon television camera.

Figure 2-14.　A. Olympus teaching attachment. B. ACMI teaching attachment.

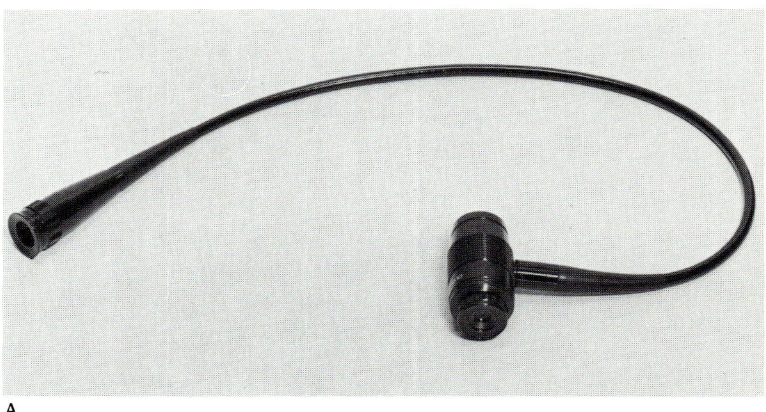

A

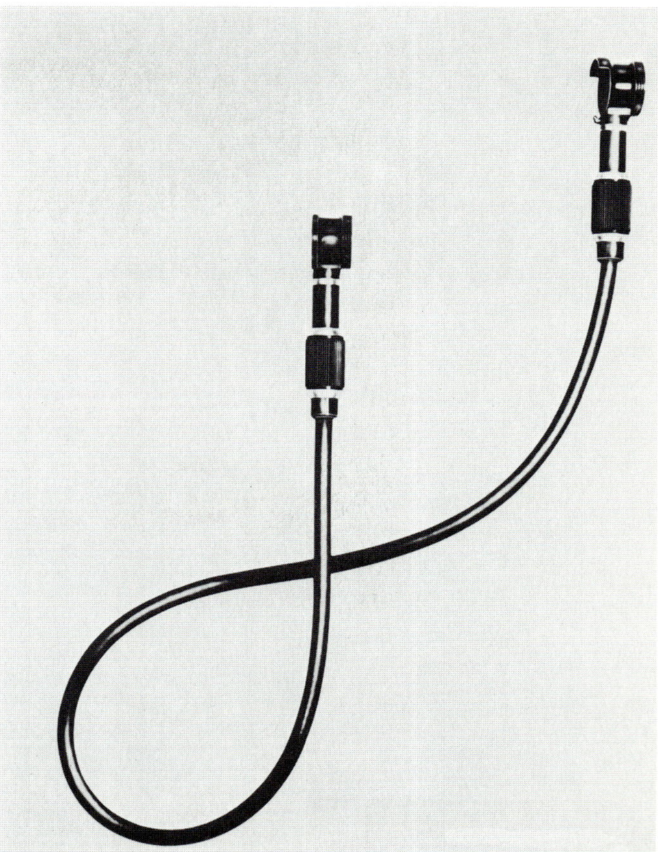

B

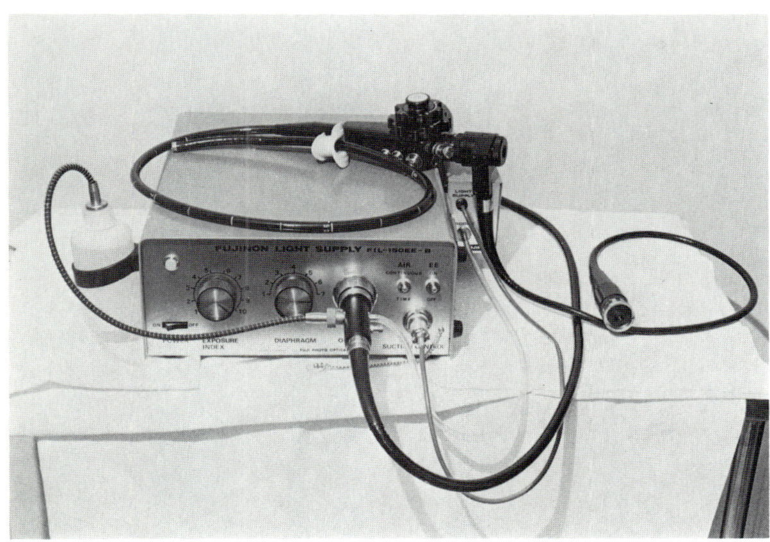

Figure 2-15.   *The Fujinon light source, panendoscope, and teaching attachment.*

CYTOLOGY BRUSHES.   Specially designed cytology brushes retrieve mucosal or surface fragments for evidence of malignant cells. To avoid loss of tissue as the brush is brought up the biopsy channel, the brush may be passed within a plastic catheter; after the brushing it may be drawn up inside the plastic catheter; the brush and catheter are then brought out so that the tissue obtained remains intact.

SUTURE REMOVAL FORCEPS.   This forceps (see Fig. 2-19) has a unique design that permits a cutting edge to slip under suture material in order to cut through it. The end of the suture can then be grasped and pulled out. Although most sutures cause no trouble, occasional ulcerations are found in association with sutures; these should definitely be removed.

OTHER ACCESSORIES.   Other very specialized devices have been developed, but they are used less frequently. Submucosal injections can

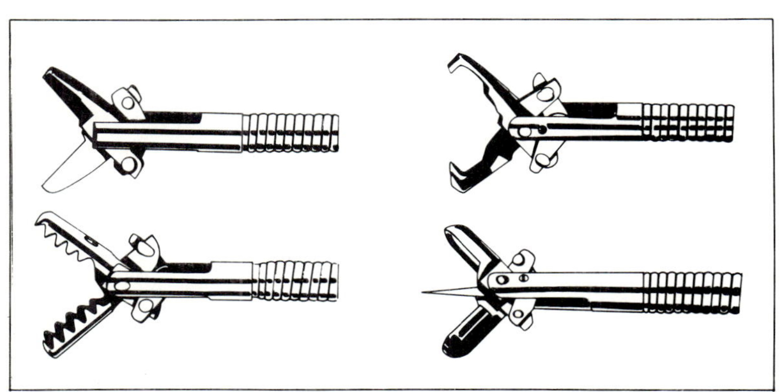

Figure 2-16.   *A variety of forceps tips.*

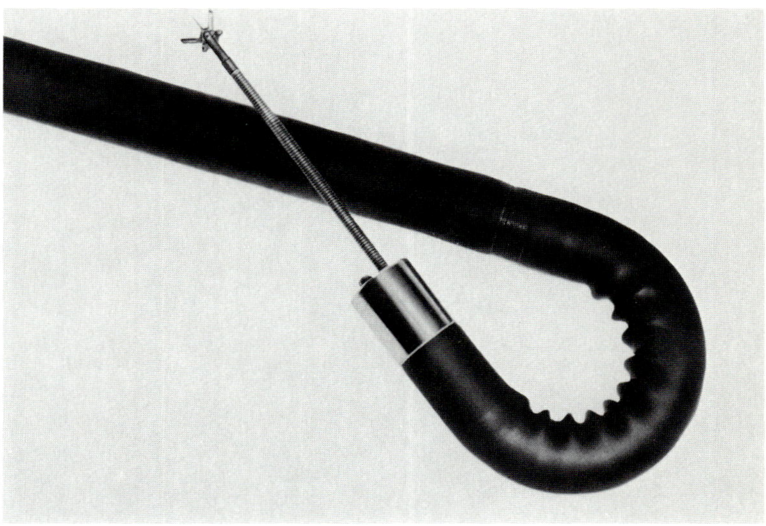

Figure 2-17. *A bayonet forceps protruding through the biopsy channel of an ACMI panendoscope.*

Figure 2-18. *The hot biopsy forceps. The electrical lead to the electrocoagulation unit is attached to the handle.*

be made with a needle attached to a catheter. These needles are designed to mark specific areas by dye injection or to control bleeding by injecting epinephrine. Esophageal varices may also be sclerosed with this needle by skilled endoscopists.

Wire baskets have been designed for the retrieval of foreign bodies and the removal of polyps excised in the stomach or colon. The open wire basket is retracted into a plastic catheter that is then inserted down the biopsy channel. When the wire is pushed through, the basket opens in much the same fashion as the polypectomy snare will open.

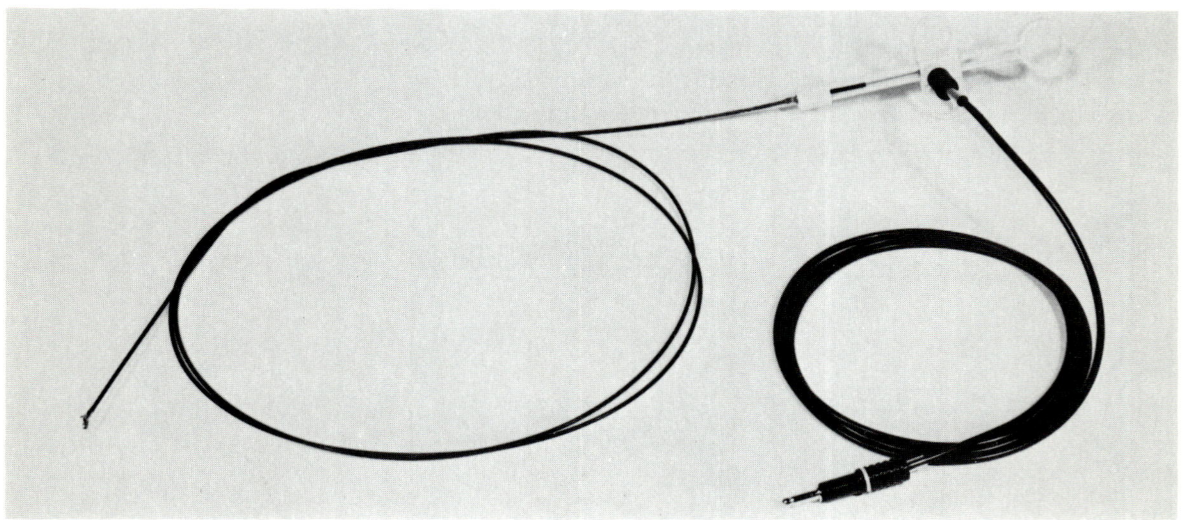

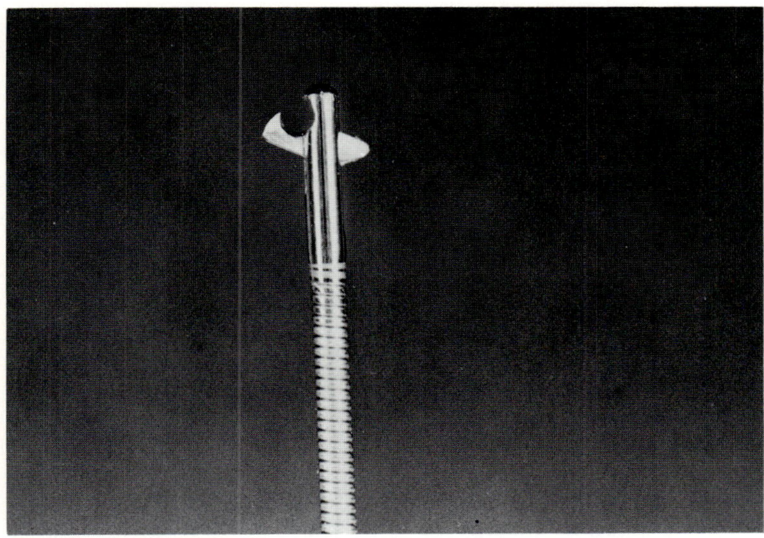

Figure 2-19.   The tip of the suture removal forceps.

A calibration catheter is available that is measured off at its tip by six 2-mm bands. This permits accurate measurement in situ of a polyp of ulcer size, and an objective evaluation of change in size at a subsequent study.

There are several devices that are specifically involved with colonoscopy. Both external and internal stiffeners—to overcome bowing of the colonoscope in the sigmoid—are available for use. These stiffeners are not usually required, however, and should be avoided since they increase the risk of the procedure and may damage the instrument. The internal stiffener is basically piano wire covered in plastic or Teflon tubing. It is inserted in the biopsy channel to reduce the flexibility of the colonoscope through the sigmoid region. The external stiffener must be in place on the proximal end of the colonoscope before intubation; it is advanced into the rectum and sigmoid colon only under fluoroscopic control.

There are many polypectomy snares (see Fig. 2-20) that are primarily used to remove polyps from the colon, but may also be used for removal of polyps in the stomach or duodenum, or for taking "jumbo" biopsies of gastric mucosa. The choice of polypectomy snare depends to a certain extent on the electrocoagulation unit used, and on the individual's experience with various types of snares, such as the single wire or braided wire types.

CARE AND MAINTENANCE OF INSTRUMENTS

Prior to the use of any endoscope, the operating mechanisms should be checked. The control knob should be rotated to be sure of a good re-

Figure 2-20.   Olympus polypectomy snares.

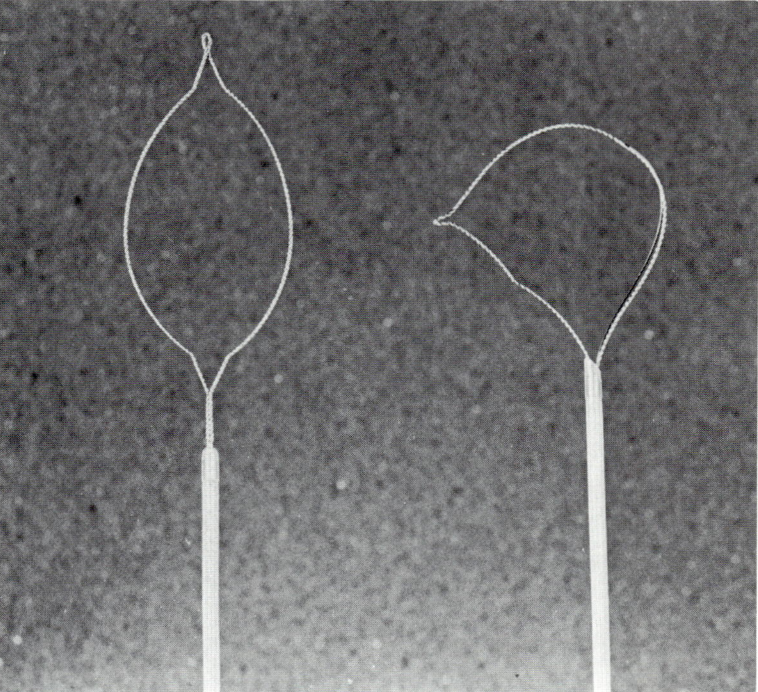

sponse at the tip. The locking mechanism should be put into place and tested. If there is a forceps-raising lever, this should be moved into both the up and the down positions. The optic system should be evaluated for adequacy of light. The bundle should be checked to determine whether a large number of fibers has been broken, and the objective lens should not show evidence of water leakage. The eyepiece should be focused properly.

Immediately following the examination, a thorough mechanical cleansing of the shaft of the endoscope and its channel should be done. A detergent solution is most effective for this purpose. This solution, followed by a water rinse, can be suctioned up the biopsy channel and then through the channel of the cord connecting the endoscope to the light source. This will flush out debris and reduce the bacterial flora.

Sterilization by the various heat modes is, of course, out of the question. If sterilization is required, it must be done by means of ethylene oxide. Gas sterilization puts the endoscope out of use for 48 hours, however, since there must be adequate aeration after the sterilization period before the instrument can be introduced into a patient.

All endoscopes may be disinfected with appropriate solutions, such as certain iodophors or glutaraldehyde. This can be accomplished by submersion of the instrument in a disinfectant such as Cidex for a period of 10 to 20 minutes. Following disinfection, the instrument must be rinsed well and thoroughly air-dried. Disinfection does not destroy the hepatitis-B virus, but there has been no documented instance of transmission of the hepatitis-B virus via endoscopic examination.

Instruments such as biopsy forceps and cytology brushes are difficult to clean, but on account of the risk of transmission of infection, these devices should be steam-sterilized and kept in a transparent bag so that they can be easily identified. Catheters for ERCP as well as polypectomy loops may be steam-sterilized after appropriate cleaning. The channels for both of these catheters can be cleaned by suctioning detergent solution through them. They can then be air-dried by further suction and sent for sterilization.

It is obvious that the half-life of an endoscope and its accessory equipment will be much greater if it is owned and employed by only one individual than if several examiners use the instrument. In the latter situation, the endoscopy assistant should be thoroughly versed in instrument maintenance, and should be permitted to inform doctors of deficiencies in their handling of instruments and equipment.

SELECTED READINGS

Berci, G. *Endoscopy*. New York: Appleton-Century-Crofts, 1976.

Boyce, H.W., Jr., and Palmer, E.D. *Technique of Clinical Gastroenterology*. Springfield, Ill.: Charles C Thomas, 1975.

Cotton, B., and Williams, B. *Practical Gastrointestinal Endoscopy*. St. Louis: Blackwell Scientific Publications, 1980.

Salmon, R.R. *Fibre-Optic Endoscopy*. London: Pitman Medical, 1974.

Schiller, K.F.R. Endoscopy. *Clin. Gastroenterol.* 7:553, 1978.

Schiller, K.F.R., and Salmon, R.R. *Modern Topics in Gastrointestinal Endoscopy*. London: William Heinemann, 1976.

CHAPTER 3

UPPER GASTROINTESTINAL ENDOSCOPY

For those who have worked with the rigid instruments available in the "good old days" of gastrointestinal endoscopy, the introduction of the fiberoptic endoscope completely changed the approach to upper gastrointestinal endoscopy. No longer was it necessary to compartmentalize the upper gastrointestinal tract into esophagus and stomach (the duodenum, of course, being out of sight). It was once necessary to insert a rigid hollow esophagoscope for examination of the esophagus and then remove it to be replaced by a semirigid gastroscope for examination of the stomach; it is now taken for granted that with fiberoptic instrumentation, all mucosal surfaces of the esophagus, stomach, and the duodenum as far as the ligament of Treitz can be examined completely. Moreover this examination can be carried out in less than 15 minutes by experienced physicians, with little or no morbidity. In addition to a complete endoscopic survey of the upper gastrointestinal tract, it is now common practice to photograph abnormalities, to obtain material for histologic examination, and to proceed with a variety of therapeutic maneuvers in the esophagus, stomach, or duodenum. This diagnostic breakthrough has preempted, in several circumstances, the barium examination of the upper gastrointestinal tract as the primary or definitive study.

INSTRUMENT AND ACCESSORIES

In 1958, Hirschowitz, Curtis, Peters, and Pollard introduced a new gastroscope called the fiberscope. Their original instrument was a side-viewing endoscope that followed the traditional design of the semiflexible prism gastroscope. The momentum toward the redesign and improvement of the fiberoptic endoscope shifted to Japan where there was a pressing need to develop a technique for the early diagnosis of stomach cancer, a disease that accounted for the majority of cancer deaths in that country. The side-viewing gastroscope did not allow visualization of the esophagus, so a short instrument was designed to view the esophagus by means of an end-on or forward-viewing esophagoscope. It was then apparent that this short fiberoptic esophagoscope could be lengthened to accomplish an examination of the esophagus, stomach, and duodenum with the one instrument. This research culminated in the presently widely used forward-viewing fiberoptic panendoscope.

There are currently four major manufacturers* in the United States marketing fiberoptic panendoscopes for examination of the upper gastrointestinal tract. The design of the instrument has been more or less standardized as the engineers have learned what does and does not work in clinical practice. The choice of instrument depends on the quality of the fiber bundle, the availability of service from the manufacturer and, to some extent, the price of endoscopic accessory equipment and light source (rather than the actual superiority of design of one panendoscope over the other). To describe each instrument manufactured by the companies listed below would be pointless since modifications of design are introduced every year or two, and if enough modifications have been made, a new model with a new label (such as GIF-D3, GIF-Q, TLX or FDS) is introduced.

The general design for a panendoscope for the examination of the upper gastrointestinal tract includes an instrument measuring approximately 120 cm in length, with an outer diameter of 11 to 13 mm (see Fig. 3-1A,B). It will have a forward-viewing optical system that provides an angle of view of at least 70 degrees, and an adjustable focus that permits a depth field of 3 mm to infinity. The tip of the instrument will bend up to approximately 180 degrees and down to 80 degrees, with a right and left turn of approximately 100 degrees (see Fig. 3-2). All instruments have a channel for the suction of air and fluid; the channel also allows for passage of biopsy forceps, catheter, or cytology brush. An elevator may also raise the forceps as it protrudes through the tip of the instrument. There must be a channel to insufflate air into the stomach, and to allow water to wash the objective lens so that mucus and blood will not obscure vision.

In general, the authors have found that one-handed manipulation of the controls allows for the most satisfactory examination technique. Therefore, the instrument with knobs that can be adjusted by the fingers of the left hand (as they reach over the handle of the instrument) provides the most suitable design (see Fig. 3-3). The left hand thus controls the motion of the tip, the insufflation of air or water, and the use of suction, allowing the right hand freedom to insert forceps or cytology brush through the channel opening or to move the shaft of the instrument as needed.

There are other instruments that offer certain advantages, but at the sacrifice of some important features. For example, a pediatric fiberscope, the outer diameter of which measures 10 mm, has all the

---

*The five equipment manufacturers and suppliers are as follows: American Cytoscope Makers, Inc. (Stamford, Connecticut); Olympus Corporation of America (New Hyde Park, New York); Fujinon Optical, Inc. (Scarsdale, New York); Pentax Precision Instrument Corporation (Norwood, New Jersey).

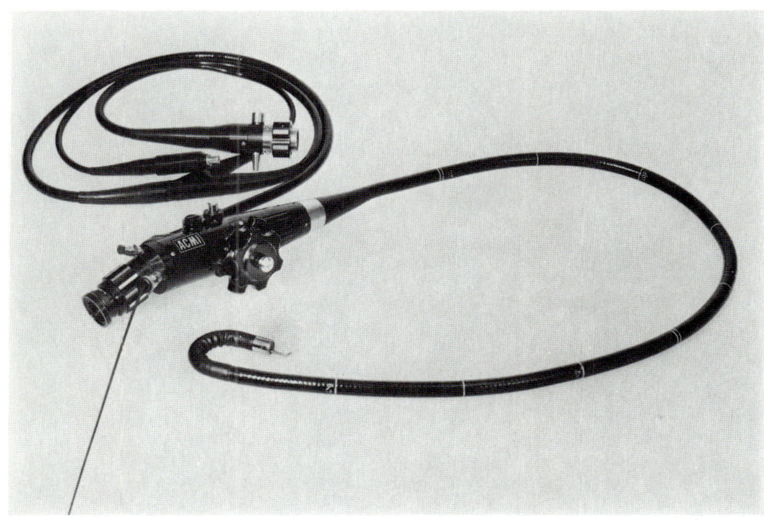

A

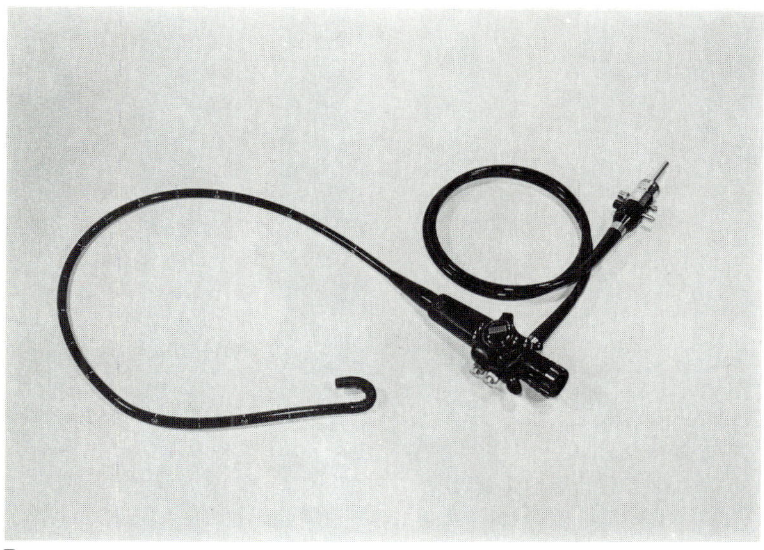

B

Figure 3-1. A. The ACMI panendoscope. B. The Olympus GIF-Q panendoscope.

design features of the larger diameter endoscope, but provides less light because of the smaller light guide bundles (although this can be compensated for by a stronger light source). It also requires a smaller biopsy forceps. This primarily pediatric instrument may be very useful in adult patients, however, who are elderly or who have narrowing of the esophageal lumen or pylorus. Indeed, this instrument can be used in well-motivated patients without any premedication at all. Moreover, it allows reasonably good visualization of the hypo-

Figure 3-2.   The tip mobility of the Olympus GIF-D3.

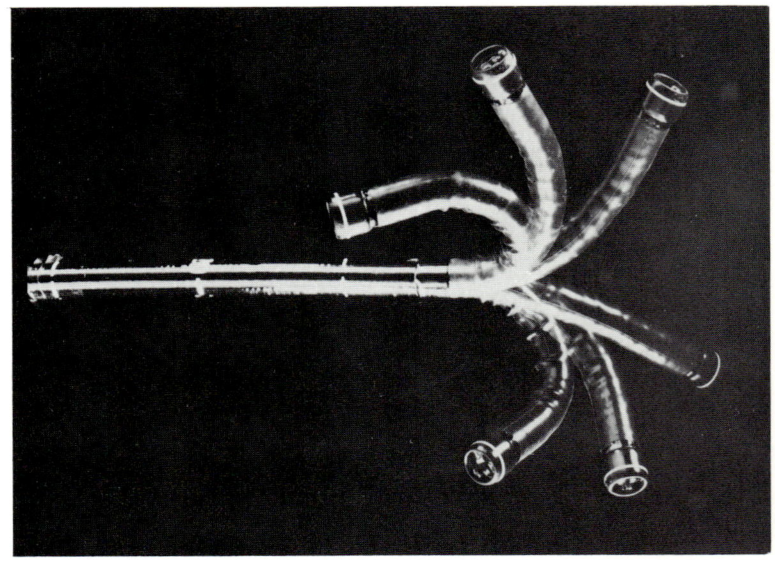

Figure 3-3.   Hand position for manipulating controls.

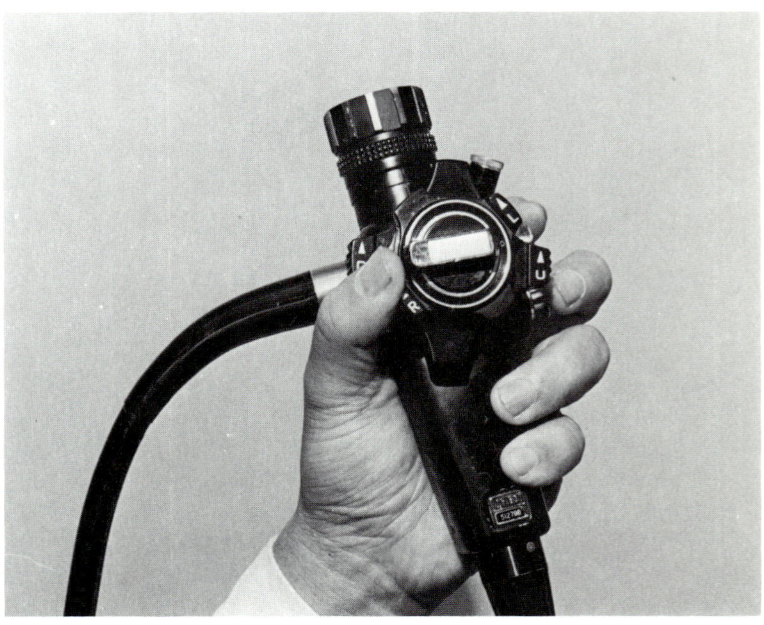

pharyngeal area as well as of the epiglottis and the vocal cords. Its increased flexibility becomes a disadvantage for the beginner in that one can get lost in the stomach when the instrument turns round on itself. It would not be surprising, however, if a smaller caliber instrument gradually replaced the present standard endoscopes for routine diagnostic study (see Fig. 3-4).

Another instrument that will be described more fully in the discussion on endoscopic retrograde cholangiopancreatography is the side-viewing gastroduodenoscope (see Fig. 6-1). This instrument, designed primarily to allow cannulation of the papilla of Vater, has certain advantages in the examination of the stomach and duodenum. First, the instrument is of smaller caliber than the forward-viewing instrument, measuring about 11 mm in diameter. Additionally, the side-viewing design permits closer inspection of the fundic and cardiac areas when the instrument is turned upon itself. It also allows better visualization of the lesser curvature of the antrum, particularly in a prominent J-type stomach. Insertion into the duodenum is not as easily accomplished, but the fornices of the duodenal bulb are visualized to a much greater extent than possible with the forward-viewing instrument. Of course it allows a direct view of the ampullary area, which is seen tangentially at best with the forward-viewing endoscope. This side-viewing gastroduodenoscope is thus a useful instrument to have in those instances when there is some question that complete visualiza-

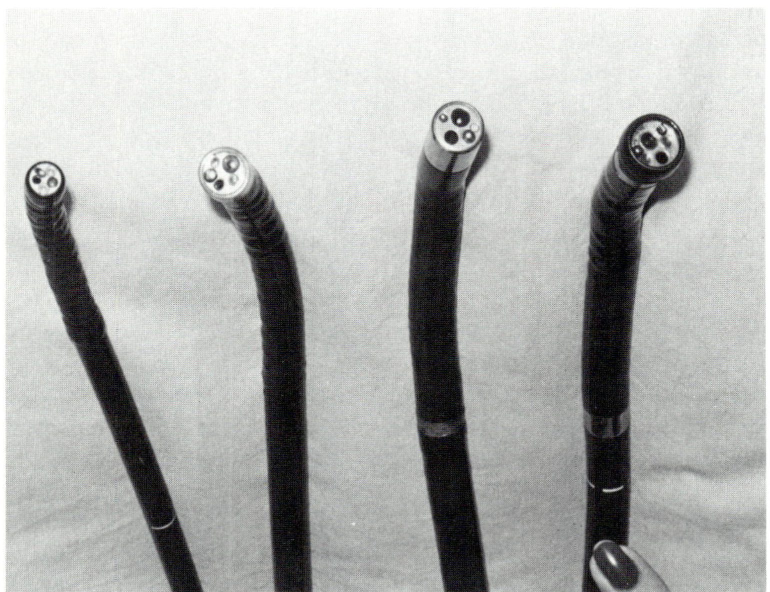

Figure 3-4. An array of panendoscope tips of small and large diameter.

tion of the stomach or duodenum was accomplished because of anatomic variation.

INDICATIONS, CONTRAINDICATIONS, AND COMPLICATIONS

Indications

Upper gastrointestinal panendoscopy is probably employed most often to explain radiologic changes of a dubious nature, or to define more exactly the nature of an x-ray finding in the esophagus, stomach, or duodenum. It is general practice, except in patients with acute gastrointestinal hemorrhage, that a barium study of the upper gastrointestinal tract precedes the endoscopic examination. The barium study can of course be done with complete safety, reduced cost, and minimal discomfort to the patient. With the new small caliber instrumentation, however, safety and discomfort are not overriding considerations, and in some other countries the cost of endoscopy is the same as or less than a barium study. Some patients prefer endoscopic intubation to barium ingestion and x-ray exposure.

Another indication for endoscopy is the examination of the patient who has persistent symptoms after a negative upper gastrointestinal series. As many as 20 percent of these patients may have positive findings by endoscopy, although perhaps in only half do the endoscopic findings contribute to the patient's symptomatology. The authors find that those patients in whom a definitive diagnosis is finally made endoscopically (and who were previously carried as functional or neurotic patients) are most appreciative of the endoscopic technique.

Obtaining tissue for histologic examination is an important example of the need for endoscopy of the upper gastrointestinal tract. This procedure is usually done when there is evidence from an upper gastrointestinal series of neoplasm of the esophagus or stomach, or of ulceration of the stomach. Under certain circumstances, however, histologic documentation of esophagitis, gastritis, or duodenitis may also be necessary. In addition to obtaining tissue by biopsy, direct brushing of a lesion for cytology may be done.

Postgastrectomy patients with upper gastrointestinal symptoms may need panendoscopy because radiologic interpretation is usually difficult in the postoperative stomach. Stomach irregularities can best be evaluated by direct visualization.

Acute bleeding from the upper gastrointestinal tract is most accurately diagnosed by panendoscopy, and this procedure should be done within 24 hours of hospitalization. The topic will be covered in detail in a subsequent chapter.

Ordinarily the finding of a duodenal ulcer by barium-contrast examination is not an indication for endoscopy. When the radiologic finding is equivocal, however, duodenoscopy is needed for accurate diagnosis. With the patient's completely informed consent, clinical research, when testing the effectiveness of one drug or another in the healing of duodenal ulcer, requires positive duodenoscopic identification of the ulcer in addition to progress duodenoscopy to confirm the healing or persistence of the ulcer. It may be necessary to prove the presence of a duodenal ulcer by endoscopy when gastric surgery is considered.

Of course peroral endoscopy lends itself to various therapeutic maneuvers that may be carried out at the initial endoscopic examination. Pedunculate polyps of the esophagus, stomach, or duodenum may be removed by the experienced and skillful endoscopist utilizing electrocoagulation snare technique. Dilatation of esophageal strictures may be done with the fiberoptic esophagoscope. Removal of foreign bodies from the esophagus, stomach, or duodenum can also be accomplished by peroral fiberendoscopy. The value of endoscopic electrocoagulation of bleeding sites in the upper gastrointestinal tract is currently being investigated, and may ultimately be indicated in specific situations.

Contraindications

The traditional contraindications for peroral endoscopy with the semiflexible instrument simply do not apply to fiberoptic methodology. One must be aware that although cervical kyphosis, anterior osteophytic proliferation of the cervical spine, and Zenker's diverticulum represent potential areas of danger, the presence of any of these anatomic impediments does not absolutely prevent fiberoptic endoscopy. Moreover, it is unlikely that the flexible instrument would in any way compromise the status of an aneurysm of the thoracic or abdominal aorta. An esophageal stricture can be dilated prior to endoscopy, although marked pyloric stenosis may prevent examination of the duodenum. Recent myocardial infarction and serious infections do not, of themselves, constitute a contraindication to flexible endoscopy if the diagnosis to be established—usually the cause or site of bleeding—influences the therapeutic program sufficiently to outweigh the risks involved.

Complications

The major complications of upper gastrointestinal endoscopy are (1) perforation, (2) bleeding, (3) cardiopulmonary accidents, (4) medication reaction, and (5) infections.

Perforation of the esophagus usually occurs in the cervical region, and in elderly patients who have degenerative spine disease with anterior spurring. Perforation of the mid- or distal esophagus is usually the result of biopsy or trauma to an area of stricture or severe inflammatory change. Perforation of the stomach is actually more common, and comprises about 60 percent of all reported perforations.

The incidence of significant bleeding as a complication is actually quite low, having been reported as 0.3 cases per 1000 endoscopic examinations. A Mallory-Weiss tear, however, has been reported following esophagoscopy.

Cardiac arrhythmia and aspiration pneumonitis are not infrequent complications, but rarely result in mortality. Aspiration is often a result of retention of gastric contents such as may occur in bleeding patients, in patients with topical anesthesia of the pharynx, and in cases of obtundity of the patient due to premedication. With the increasing use of intravenous diazepam, respiratory arrest is being recognized more frequently; it is probably the most common pulmonary complication. If patients are monitored by electrocardiography during upper gastrointestinal endoscopy, fleeting irregularities of cardiac rhythm, including tachycardia, bradycardia, and premature contractions may be seen in a large percentage of patients, particularly those with preexisting heart disease.

The complications of premedication are often due to marked obtundity in elderly or cirrhotic patients who cannot metabolize even small doses of meperidine or phenobarbital. Atropine-like drugs may induce tachycardia or precipitate urinary obstruction in elderly men. Phlebitis at the site of intravenous injection of diazepam is not uncommon. Anaphylactic reactions to topical anesthetics are rare, but they can be fatal.

Transient bacteremia may occur, but no case of endocarditis related to upper gastrointestinal endoscopy has been reported. Patients with prosthetic heart valves, however, should be protected by prophylactic antibiotics. There has been no reported incidence of transmission of hepatitis-B virus related to an endoscopic procedure. Mechanical cleansing of the instrument with soap, water, and alcohol appears to be adequate to prevent serious infection, but disinfection with such agents as glutaraldehyde would add an additional measure of safety.

PREPARATION

The most important aspect of preparation of the patient is the preliminary discussion of the procedure and its possible complications. A well-motivated patient will give the doctor the kind of cooperation that will make for a smooth and orderly study. The patient should be assured that the instrument is neither rigid nor metallic but flexible, and can be passed into the esophagus without any effort on his part. The patient should be informed that gagging will be minimized by topical anesthesia, and that it is not necessary to "swallow" the instrument. Although the risk is miniscule, the patient should be told that a perforation of the esophagus or stomach is possible, and that he or she will be under observation for a period of time after the procedure. The authors believe that it is unfair, however, to test the psychologic defenses of the patient by describing in detail the dire consequences of this untoward event (that is, perforation).

Upper gastrointestinal endoscopy for diagnostic purposes is basically an outpatient procedure. Hospitalization is not required for peroral endoscopy. The procedure should be done in a room specifically designed for this purpose. Under special circumstances, however, it may be done in a patient's hospital room or in an intensive care facility.

It is important that the endoscopy assistant also gain rapport with the patient. The assistant is not there merely to hold the head of the patient, but to be part of the team. The assistant should project a sense of serenity, confidence, and control. If things do not go smoothly during the initial preparation of the patient, then the whole procedure can be jeopardized by the patient's anxiety.

The assistant should bring the patient into the room, chatting amiably at the time. The patient should be questioned to be sure that nothing has been ingested in the last 6 to 8 hours. An inquiry should be made as to whether the patient has developed a sore throat or an upper respiratory infection since last talking to the doctor. Although the patient would have been advised previously by the endoscopist about the medication that is taken first thing in the morning, it is wise for the assistant to check that these instructions have been followed. Necklaces, pendants, and earrings should be removed. All dentures and removable partial dental bridges should be taken out and put aside in a container.

The patient is given Simethicone solution. Anesthetic spray such as Cetacaine spray (Benzocaine 14%, Tetracaine Hydrochloride 2%) may be used, or the pharynx may be swabbed with 1% Tetracaine Hydrochloride or 5% Hexylcaine. Some physicians prefer just to have the patient gargle, but gargling may anesthetize the tongue and buccal mucosa, causing the patient to handle secretions poorly, and also increasing the possibility of excess dosage by the patient swallowing the anesthetic agent. If there has been a history of prior reaction to topical anesthetics, then it is best to use a solution of an antihistamine such as Diphenhydramine. When using an antihistamine solution for topical anesthesia, however, one might legitimately question the effectiveness of the agent beyond the placebo effect. Most patients expect topical anesthesia and become anxious if no effort is made to anesthetize the pharynx.

The assistant should then position the patient on the examining table. The standard position is the left lateral decubitus. It is possible to use almost any position for flexible peroral endoscopy, including sitting, supine, or right lateral decubitus. The authors have found that the left lateral position provides the most comfort for the patient (see Fig. 3-5). The patient rests on the left shoulder with the left arm behind the back. Both thighs are flexed, the right thigh more than the left, and the right knee is used as a pivotal support so that the patient is leaning somewhat forward. The patient's head is on a pillow and the right arm may rest along the hip, or the right hand may grasp the edge of the table in front. At this point, a suitable vein is found for the intravenous injection of diazepam. It is best to position the patient prior to giving the medication, since once the patient becomes sedated it is difficult to move him from the supine position, particularly if he is overweight (and unfortunately many patients in the United States are overweight).

A narcotic preparation frequently is used for premedication. These drugs may drop blood pressure in elderly patients; the dosage should be adjusted accordingly. Anticholinergic agents are given to reduce oral secretion, but they may be omitted where tachycardia, prolonged dry mouth, and bowel distention could be a problem. Usually 2.5 to 10.0 mg of intravenous diazepam is given immediately after the patient has been positioned. The patient is carefully observed as the drug is slowly introduced. Slurred speech or horizontal nystagmus represent the endpoint of the injection. At times it is convenient to have a butterfly needle attached to a flexible catheter kept open with a syringe of

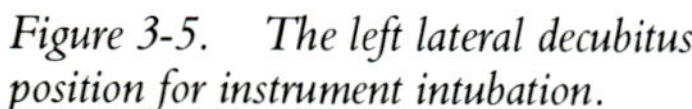

Figure 3-5.   The left lateral decubitus position for instrument intubation.

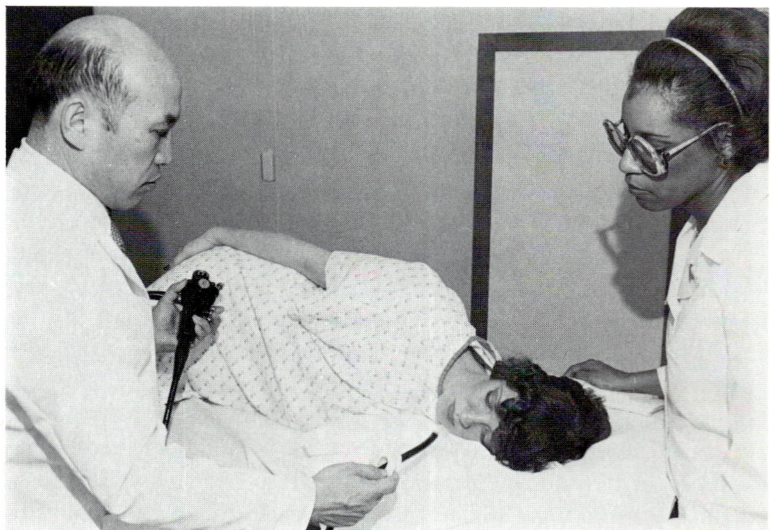

sterile saline. This allows additional injections of diazepam to be given during the course of the endoscopic procedure. Diazepam has proven to be a remarkably safe agent for the authors. Although a burning sensation may be noted with the injection of the drug, rarely has there been evidence of a subsequent phlebitis. Upper respiratory depression may occur, but this is usually counteracted by commanding the patient to breathe or by the stimulation of the procedure itself.

TECHNIQUE OF ESOPHAGOGASTRODUODENOSCOPY
Forward-Viewing Instrument

The endoscopist is now ready to proceed with the evaluation of the upper gastrointestinal tract. He or she stands facing the patient who lies on the table, which is at a comfortable height for the endoscopist. The assistant stands or sits on a high stool at the patient's head. The assistant's hand is placed at the back of the patient's head for reassurance and to prevent any reflex withdrawal as the intubation proceeds, but not to hold the head. The instrument should have been checked by the assistant before the procedure, but often the endoscopist himself will prefer to check the vital functions of the endoscope. The endoscopist turns on the power source to be sure that there is a light available, checks the air insufflation and water valve, and tests for adequacy of the suction. The knobs are turned slightly to observe the response of the tip. The endoscopist glances about to see that the camera is ready, and the teaching attachment nearby. A disposable glove is then put on the left hand, and the maneuverable portion of the tip of the instrument is covered with water-soluble jelly. The right hand grasps the shaft of the instrument by its midsection; the handle is supported by the assistant, and the tip of the instrument is grasped with the left hand as one would hold a billiard cue (see Fig. 3-6). The plastic mouthpiece must be in place on the instrument before intubation. Following intubation, the plastic mouthpiece is then brought down and placed between the patient's teeth or gingivae. In the event that the mouthpiece has not been put in place, it is always wise to have a mouthpiece that has been slit at the side so that it can be placed around the fiberscope after intubation.

An alternate method of insertion is to pass the end-viewing fiberscope, with the lateral control locked, through the plastic mouthpiece placed between the patient's teeth or gingivae (see Fig. 3-7). A finger is not inserted into the mouth during the endoscopic intubation. The tip of the scope is brought to the base of the tongue, which is pushed forward slightly. The instrument is then advanced into the hypopharynx, keeping it as much as possible in the midline. In a few patients it may be necessary to check the oral pharynx directly, to

Figure 3-6.   The insertion of the panendoscope using the fingers of the left hand to guide the instrument.

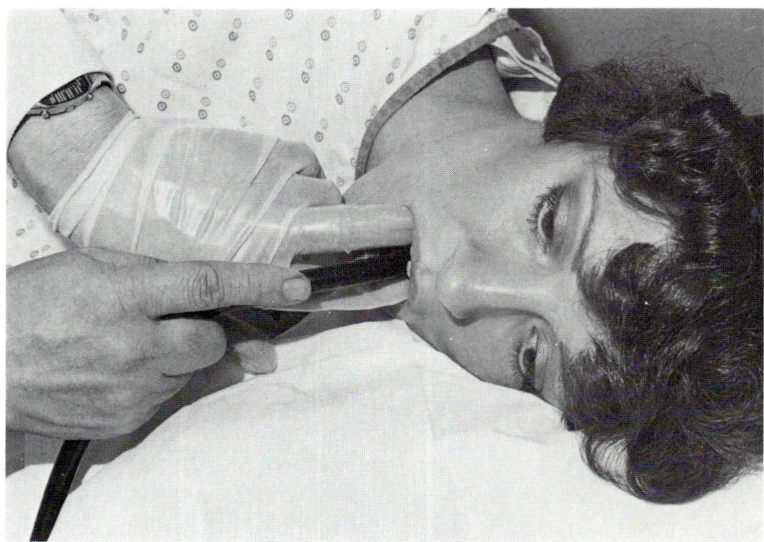

make sure that the scope is going in line with the cricopharyngeus sphincter. This type of intubation will be successful in almost all patients. The technique allows direct visualization of the intubation, and can be used to advantage with the patient who is actively bleeding.

After the instrument has passed the hypopharynx, the patient is asked only to breathe normally, and should not be burdened by a lot of

Figure 3-7.   Direct intubation with the panendoscope.

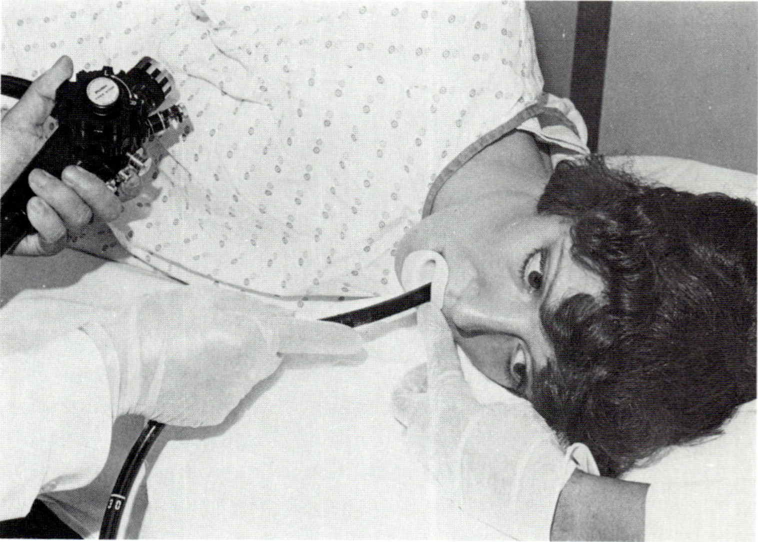

commands. Resistance will be met at the cricopharyngeus sphincter; this occurs at the 20-cm mark on the endoscope. It goes without saying that force is not used to pass this area of resistance. Some patients cannot swallow voluntarily under these circumstances, which can be very frustrating; if one observes the neck of the patient, there will be seen reflex swallowing efforts. At this point, however, the cricopharyngeus muscle will generally relax and intubation will proceed into the lumen of the esophagus. Sometimes the endoscope can be passed in the sitting position more readily than in the lateral decubitus position. If the standard 12-mm scope fails, then the smaller caliber lateral-viewing or pediatric instrument should almost certainly succeed (see Fig. 3-8).

Once the cricopharyngeus sphincter has been overcome, the instrument is then passed under direct vision to the cardia. It is assumed that a previous barium study has not demonstrated any stricture of the esophagus, but an occasional stricture may not be appreciated, or a Schatzki ring may have been overlooked. One must proceed under direct vision, therefore, to be sure that there is an adequate lumen ahead at all times. If a ring is found, it may be narrow enough to impede the progress of the instrument. The ring may be dilated by the endoscope itself. Unfortunately, the authors are aware of at least one instance where such a dilation led to a severe hemorrhage. In normal patients, the Z line of the esophagogastric mucosal junction is readily identified at 37 to 40 cm (see Fig. 3-9A), and one proceeds to the cardia where the attachment of the diaphragmatic muscles can be noted by asking the

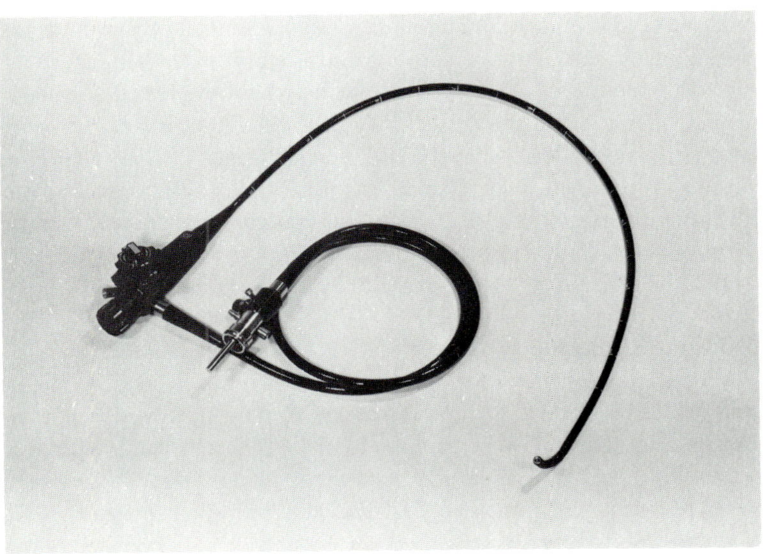

Figure 3-8.   The Olympus GIF-P2 panendoscope which allows successful intubation of almost every patient.

patient to sniff. In the presence of a hiatal hernia, the Z line will generally be above the level of 37 cm, and the herniated portion of the stomach will be at least 3 cm above the impingement of the diaphragmatic muscles on the stomach. While traversing the esophagus, it is wise to suction out secretions that are present, to avoid their aspiration.

When the stomach is entered (see Fig. 3-9B), it is usually already distended by air that has been insufflated into the esophagus. The chamber of the fundus comes into view, and secretions may be evident along the greater curvature side of the stomach. It is wise to suction these secretions as completely as possible; if the patient then retches, there will not be reflux up the esophagus and into the mouth. In patients who have fasted for 6 to 8 hours as directed, there should not be any remnants of food or other particulate matter in the stomach. If there is, it suggests either partial gastric outlet obstruction or diminished gastric peristalsis. Once the stomach has been suctioned free of liquid residual, it is then reinflated, and the intubation is carried out so that the duodenum will be reached as soon as possible. Thus no attempt is made to study any pathology encountered as the instrument moves from organ to organ. A mental note is made of any abnormality, so that it will not be overlooked on withdrawal of the instrument.

One then moves from the fundus of the stomach into the body of the stomach by turning the shaft of the scope clockwise. The landmark to be found in the body of the stomach is, of course, the angulus (see Fig. 3-9C). With the forward-viewing instrument, the angulus does not appear as prominent a landmark as with the lateral-viewing instrument. Ordinarily there is no difficulty in finding the antral segment beyond the crescentic fold that demarcates the body from the antrum. The pylorus usually comes promptly into view (see Fig. 3-9D), but occasionally in a J-shaped stomach (where the antral segment is acutely bent along the lesser curvature of the distal body of the stomach), the pylorus may be difficult to locate. By applying some torque on the shaft of the instrument in a clockwise direction, and by directing the tip somewhat to the right, however, the pylorus can then be identified. If the pylorus moves away as it is pursued, the scope should be manipulated to keep the pyloric ring in the middle of the visual field.

Insertion into the pylorus should not be difficult (see Fig. 3-9E). There is often resistance to the pressure of the tip of the endoscope, but this yields promptly in most instances. At times, however, it is not possible to easily intubate the duodenal bulb, and several approaches may be necessary. The resistance of the pylorus cannot be overcome by repeated jabbing motions, but the gate will open to steady gentle pressure. Sometimes as this pressure is applied, the endoscopist may find that the instrument is gradually being inserted to its full length. This means that the greater curvature of the stomach is being stretched out by this force. It is therefore necessary for an assistant to place counterpressure with the hand along the greater curvature of the stomach. This counterpressure will generally lead to a release of resistance, and the instrument tip pops into the duodenal bulb. Actually, the time the endoscope is stuck in the pylorus may be the best opportunity to survey the duodenal bulb, since on withdrawal of the instrument it may be difficult to maintain the endoscope in the duodenal bulb. The impasse at the pylorus can be used to advantage, therefore, and one should not rush this phase of the intubation. On occasion, the pylorus cannot be intubated; this suggests that cicatricial changes have taken place, and that there is a fixed narrowing at this point. To exclude pyloric stenosis, one should, however, give an intravenous anticholinergic agent or glucagon and observe whether this permits passage or not. Pediatric panendoscopes will rarely fail to pass the pylorus, and often allow better visualization of the duodenal bulb than the standard instrument.

Once in the duodenal bulb (see Fig. 3-9F), it is not difficult to find one's way into the descending duodenum. Again, torque on the shaft in a clockwise rotation with direction of the tip to the right will often allow the tip to fall into the descending duodenum which, after inflation, can then be surveyed with ease. Without fluoroscopic control, it is impossible to judge how far the duodenum has been traversed beyond the second portion. One can move into the third portion of the duodenum in most patients, although this is not forcibly attempted if there is resistance, since the likelihood of pathology beyond the second portion is remote. If the ligament of Treitz is to be reached, then the examination should be conducted with the patient under the fluoroscope, and the instrument palpated and manipulated through the abdominal wall in such a way as to use the effective total length of the panendoscope.

From the descending duodenum, the instrument is withdrawn and the mucosa is examined. Further penetration into the descending duodenum occurs when the scope is withdrawn, because the loop in the stomach is straightened. The circumferential folds of the duodenum are readily recognized, and should be easily flattened with instillation of air. The major papilla of the duodenum is seen on a tangential view. Once the superior angle of the duodenum is reached, the folds disappear; the mucosa of the duodenal bulb is very similar to that of the antrum. The distal bulb can be seen completely with the forward-viewing instrument, but obviously the fornices of the duodenal bulb will not be viewed.

Once the tip has been withdrawn from the duodenal bulb, the

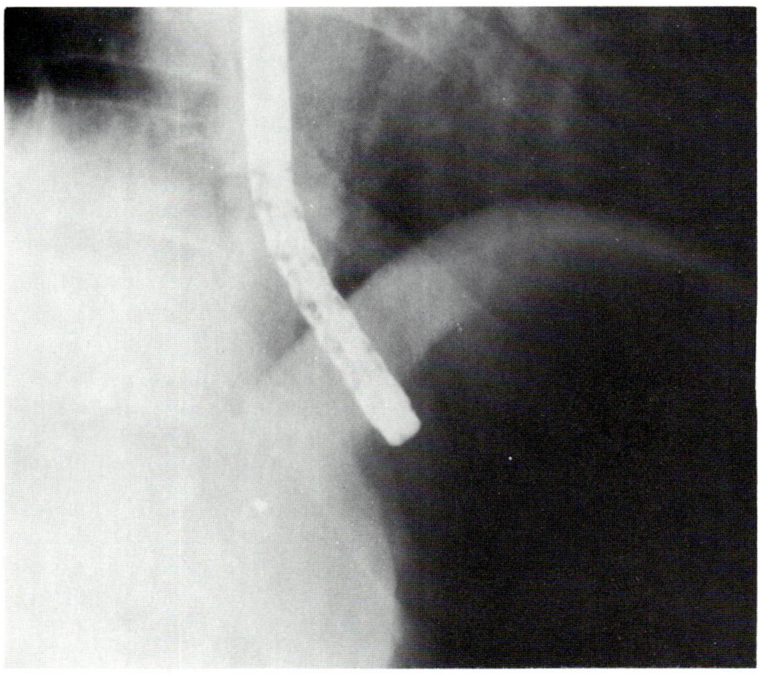

Figure 3-9.   A. The tip of the endoscope has just passed the E–G junction. B. The tip is at the high lesser curvature level of the inflated stomach. C. The tip is at the angulus. D. The pylorus is in view as the endoscope enters the antrum. E. The duodenal bulb has been intubated. F. The tip is at the apex of the bulb from which it will be bent caudad to be inserted into the descending duodenum. G. The J-turn maneuver to view the lesser curvature and cardia of the stomach. H. The U-turn maneuver along the greater curvature provides a perspective of the greater curvature, fundus, and cardia.

A

B

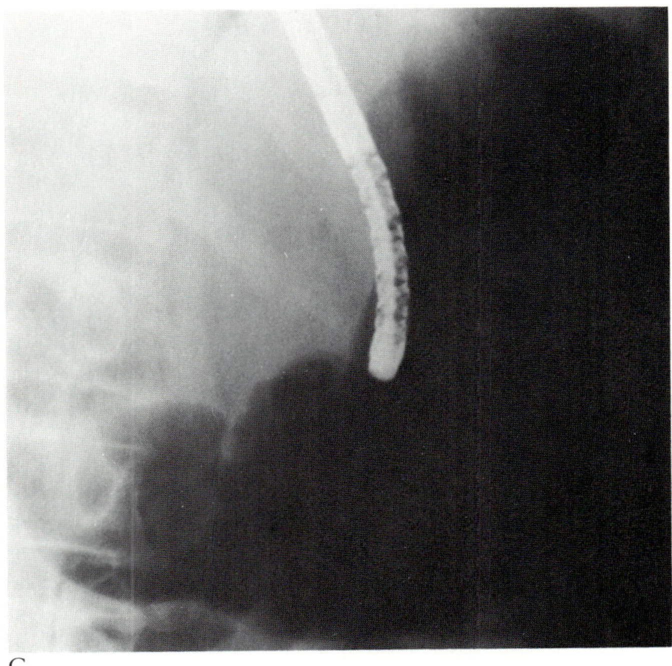

C

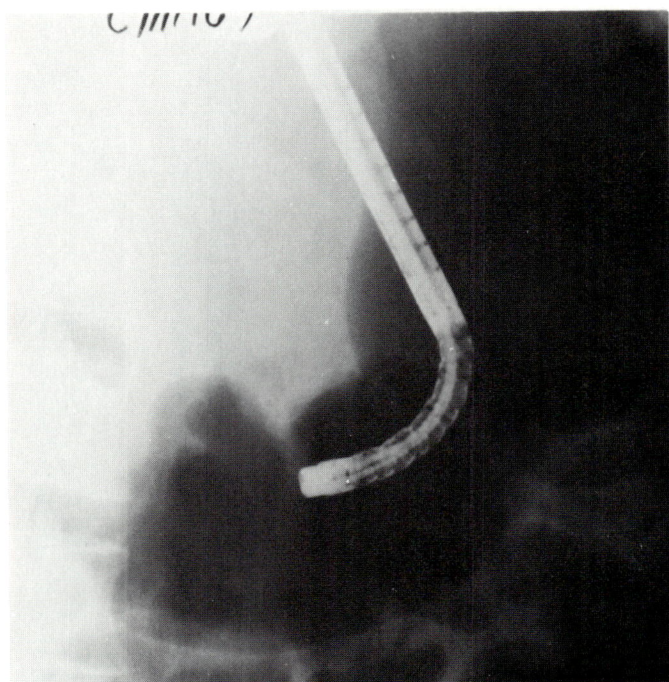

D

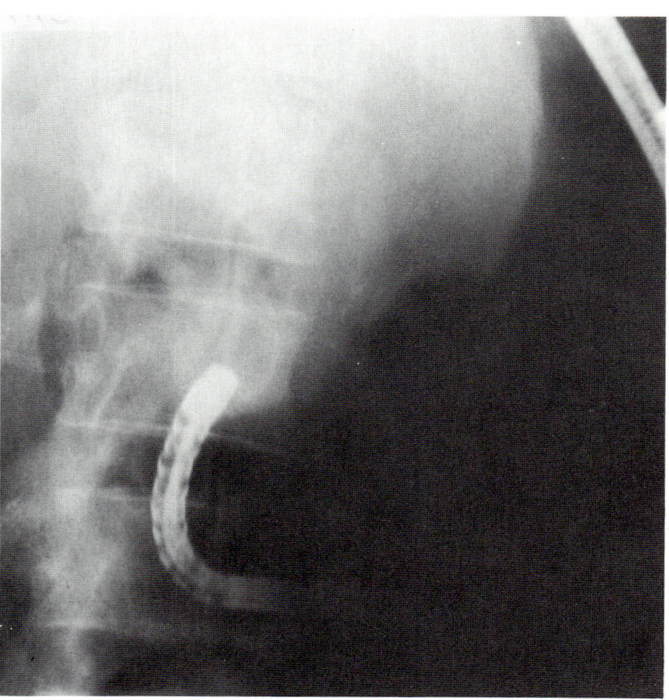

E

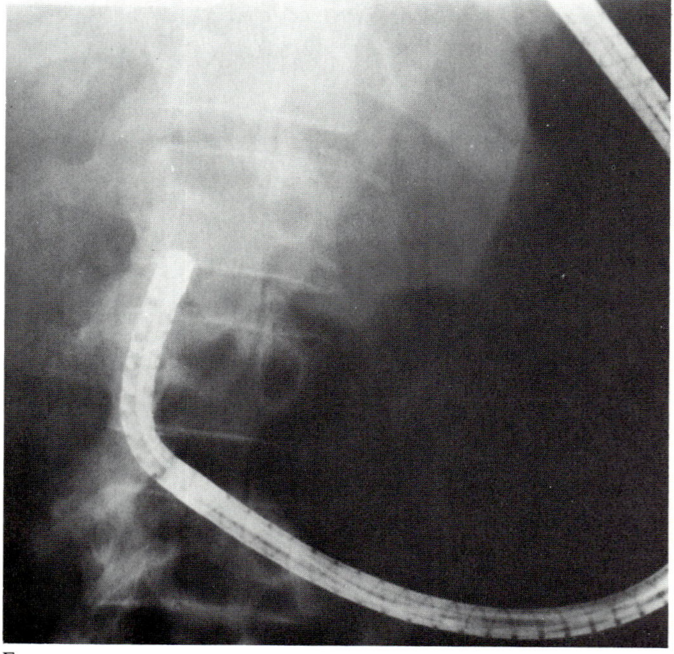

F

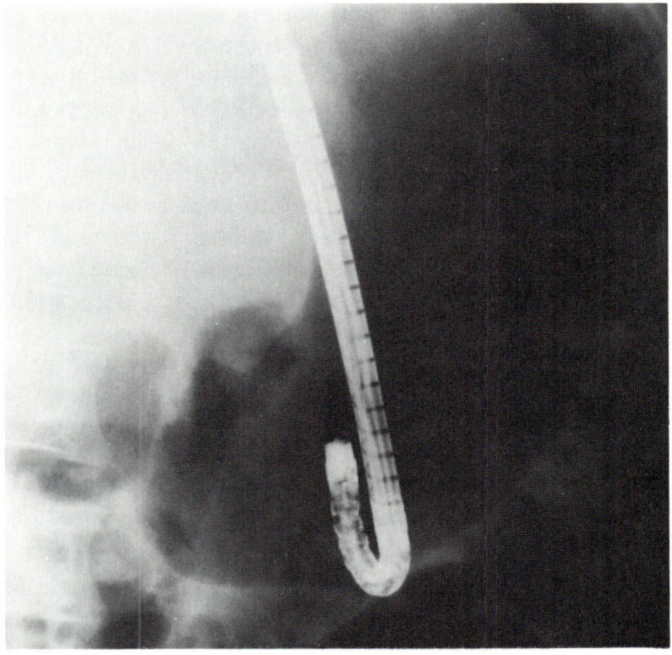

G

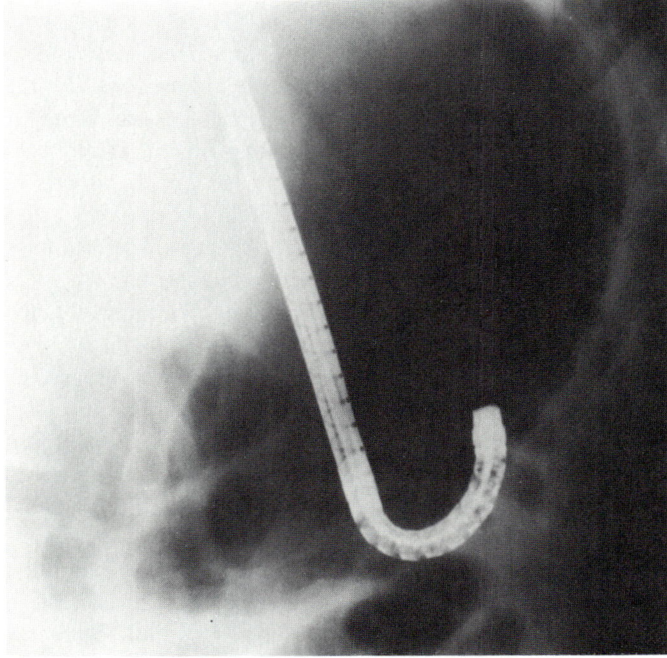

H

pylorus is again inspected, and the lesser curvature of the antrum brought into view. This is usually accomplished by waiting for peristaltic waves to move through the antrum. Occasionally in a J-type stomach, the lesser curvature of the antrum is difficult to see, and it may be necessary to move the patient into different positions to be certain that the area has been totally examined. The antrum may be brought into view when a peristaltic wave moves through. There is no problem in examining the greater curvature of the antrum, and the body of the stomach can be inflated so that the folds along the greater curvature are flattened out. The tip is moved in a circumferential manner to bring the total surface area of the body of the stomach into view.

One then brings the endoscope back up to the level of the cardia, and from that position one can generally see the greater curvature side of the fundus and some of the distal lesser curvature side. To see the cap of the fundus and the area about the cardia, it is necessary to turn the instrument on itself. To accomplish this, the endoscope is then passed to a point just proximal to the angulus. It is then flexed upward to its full extent and the endoscope is advanced, putting some clockwise torque on the instrument as the advance is made. The fundus will come into view after turning the tip to the right somewhat (see Fig. 3-9G), and the instrument will be seen emerging from the cardia, usually at the level of the 20-cm marking on the endoscope. In addition to this J-turn maneuver, the tip may be bent down and a U turn can be made along the greater curvature of the stomach (see Fig. 3-9H). Because the light is diffuse in this area, it is best to take the teaching attachment off to view the fundus completely and to examine the area around the cardia. The only blind area will be the mucosa covered by the endoscope itself. This can be uncovered by putting torque on the instrument or by instrument withdrawal, which paradoxically often brings you a closer view of the fundus and cardia. There is some concern about the possibility of impacting the tip of the endoscope into the cardia adjacent to the shaft. This can happen if the instrument is turned about too high in the stomach.

The instrument is then allowed to straighten out as it is withdrawn, once the physician is sure that the lock is off the control wheels. It will then be pulled up into the cardia, and the esophagogastric mucosal junction will be recognized once again by the appearance of the Z line. The instrument is then carefully withdrawn up the esophagus, the lumen of which can be kept open readily with gentle insufflation of air. The lumen of the esophagus should be narrower than approximately twice the diameter of the endoscope. Peristaltic waves can be readily identified traversing the esophagus, but it is rarely possible to recognize a disorder of esophageal motility by observation of esophageal peristalsis. The upper third of the esophagus should be checked for instrumental trauma, should there have been difficulty in the intubation. In the hypopharynx, it is not uncommon to get a view of the epiglottis and the vocal cords, although this is considerably easier to do with the pediatric instrument than the 12-mm one. The instrument is then completely removed and the mouthpiece is taken from the patient's mouth.

The endoscopist then directs his full attention to the patient. The patient must clear his mouth of all secretions. Once the physician is assured that there is no danger of aspiration and that the patient is sufficiently awake, it is best to have the patient sit up and allow him to belch out any air that has remained in the stomach. The patient should be observed for a few minutes in the sitting position; during this time he or she may be assured about the findings of the examination and complimented on his cooperation. The patient is brought to a bed where he or she may rest until completely recovered from the effects of the medication.

Lateral-Viewing Instrument

Due to some variation of gastric anatomy as indicated previously, it may not be possible to view completely the mucosa of the stomach, or at least to obtain a completely satisfactory examination of a lesion. For example, the lesser curvature of the antrum in a J-shaped stomach may be impossible to view completely with the forward-viewing instrument. High lesser curvature lesions may be found only with a lateral-viewing instrument, particularly in a cascade type of a stomach. A much closer inspection of the cardiac and fundic area of this type of stomach can be made with the lateral-viewing gastroscope. Moreover, the duodenal bulb may be examined in such a way as to complement the view of the forward-viewing instrument and thereby allow more complete visualization of this area. Only the lateral-viewing instrument permits a thorough inspection of the major and minor papilla of the duodenum.

The technique for passage of the lateral-viewing gastroduodenoscope is identical to that of the forward-viewing instrument. Indeed, the intubation is considerably easier because of the smaller diameter of the currently popular (1978) model, the JF-B3 from the Olympus Corporation (see Fig. 3-10). Although the distal esophagus may be visualized by angulation of the tip, this is not an ideal way to do an esophageal study. The angulus is readily identified, being a much more prominent landmark for those using this type of instrument. The pylorus is brought easily into view if the antrum is not over distended and if the tip is rotated somewhat to the right. Of course, direct intubation cannot be made with this instrument. As the tip is advanced to the pylorus, the rim of the pylorus is lost to view. A

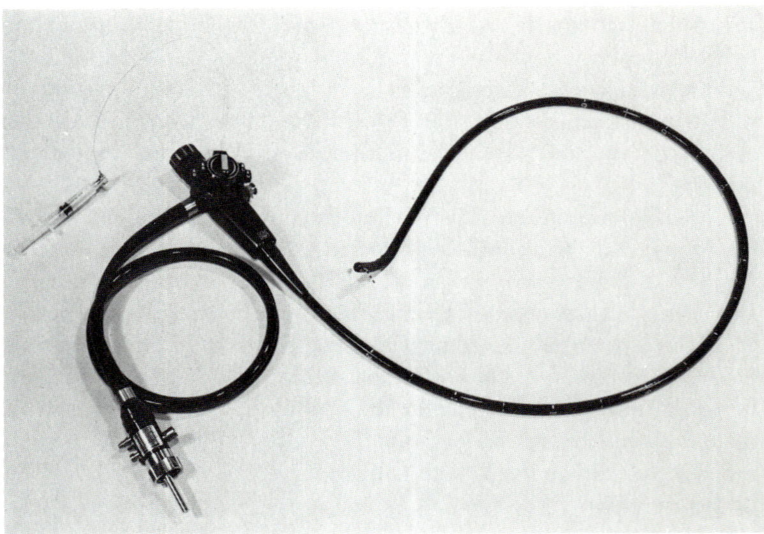

Figure 3-10.   The Olympus JF-B3 duodenoscope.

slight upward movement of the tip, accompanied by forward motion of the instrument and some clockwise torque on the shaft, will generally allow passage of the instrument into the duodenal bulb. The pylorus will yield to gentle but steady pressure. Once the bulb is entered, further clockwise rotation of the instrument with the tip slightly up will bring the endoscope into the descending duodenum. The instrument will then pass to the inferior duodenal angle, or the junction of the second and third position of the duodenum.

As the lateral-viewing duodenoscope is withdrawn, adequate inflation of the descending duodenum must be made to obtain a good look at the mucosa. The characteristic appearance of this area is that of a series of circumferential folds. There is usually active peristalsis through the descending duodenum, and if the papilla is to be located readily, glucagon or an anticholinergic agent such as propanthilene or tridihexethyl chloride must be given intravenously. About the midportion of the descending duodenum on the medial wall, a vertical fold will usually be identified; by following this fold toward the superior angle of the duodenum, the papilla may be found. The papilla may be only a few centimeters from the apex of the bulb, or it may be located on occasion in the distal portion of the descending duodenum, or anywhere between. The papilla varies in size and shape as well as position. It may appear as a prominent nipple or may be barely discernible from the surrounding mucosa. If intravenous glucagon is given, the shape of the papilla may change with relaxation of the ampullary musculature.

As the instrument is withdrawn into the bulb, one must be careful that the endoscope does not fall out into the stomach; some counter pressure must therefore be applied as the bulb is inspected. Bending of the tip as well as axial rotation of the instrument itself will allow examination of the proximal portion of the duodenal bulb, the area that is not examined with a forward-viewing duodenoscope.

On withdrawal of the instrument from the duodenum into the stomach, an examination of the antrum with particular attention to the lesser curvature is carried out. Again the body of the stomach may be examined completely with circumferential rotation of the tip. The greater curvature of the stomach is seen as the instrument is withdrawn to the upper third of the stomach. At this point, the tip is retroflexed, and the fundus and cardia area can be completely examined without difficulty. For a closer examination of the cardia area, this instrument can also be retroverted, with the cardia and the cap of the fundus brought into proximity. The instrument is then straightened out and withdrawn, with inspection of the distal esophagus.

SELECTED READINGS

Cotton, P.B.   Upper Gastrointestinal Endoscopy. In L.M. Nyhus and C. Wastell, *Surgery of the Stomach and Duodenum*. Boston: Little, Brown, 1977. P. 149.

Mandelstam, P., et al.   Complications associated with esophagogastroduodenoscopy and with esophageal dilation: An analysis of the 1974 ASGE Survey. *Gastrointest. Endosc.* 23:16, 1976.

Morrissey, J.F.   Progress in gastroenterology, gastrointestinal endoscopy. *Gastroenterology* 62:1241, 1972.

Salmon, P.R.   *Fiberoptic Endoscopy*. London: Pitman, 1974.

Schuman, B.M.   The gastroscopic yield from the negative upper gastrointestinal series. *Gastrointest. Endosc.* 19:79, 1972.

Sugawa, C., and Walt, A.J.   *Scope and Technique of Upper Gastrointestinal Endoscopy*. (Movie) From the Motion Picture Library, American College of Surgeons. Danbury, Conn.: Davis & Geck, Distributors, 1976. 23 minutes.

Waye, J.D.   The current status of flexible fiberoptic endoscopy. *Mt. Sinai J. Med. (N.Y.)* 42:1, 1975.

Wolff, W.I., and Shinya, H.   Modern Endoscopy of the Alimentary Tract. In *Current Problems in Surgery*. Chicago: Year Book, January 1974.

CHAPTER 4

UPPER GASTROINTESTINAL ENDOSCOPIC FINDINGS

ESOPHAGUS

Neoplasms of the Esophagus

ESOPHAGEAL CANCER.   Endoscopy should be performed in all patients suspected of having esophageal cancer, to establish a tissue diagnosis and to determine accurately the orad limit of the lesion.

Carcinoma of the esophagus occurs most frequently as a fungating, obstructing, and occasionally ulcerating growth (see Plates 1 and 2). A stenosing carcinoma may be difficult to differentiate from a benign stricture. Multiple forceps biopsies, cytologic brushing, or large particle biopsy from nodular areas and from the stricture itself are often necessary to obtain tumor cells. Most of the cancers involving the esophagogastric junction are adenocarcinoma of gastric origin. The pediatric endoscope can be passed through the narrowed area, and the turnaround maneuver may then show the lesion arising from the cardia.

BENIGN TUMOR.   Benign submucosal tumors such as leiomyomas, lipomas, and neurofibromas are seen as round, smooth, polypoid lesions with occasional central ulceration. Forceps biopsy almost always shows normal esophageal tissue (see Plate 3).

Esophageal Varices

With portal hypertension, vessels in the submucosal plexus of the esophageal mucosa increase in size and become dilated. These dilated veins are, in fact, esophageal varices. Typically these varices appear as longitudinal, tortuous, and beaded mucosal elevations extending from the mid- to distal esophagus, and often into the cardia of the stomach (see Plate 4). The varices may be off-gray or blue in color, but frequently do not differ from the surrounding mucosa. Only one varix may be apparent, or the varices may be restricted to the area of the cardia.

A blood clot or erosion on a varix is a sign of recent bleeding. If the examination is done during active bleeding, oozing or spurting of blood may be seen (Plate 42). Varices can be differentiated from esophageal folds endoscopically by flattening the folds during air insufflation, or by demonstrating distention of the veins when the patient performs a Valsalva maneuver.

Hiatal Hernia

The most common type of esophageal hiatal hernia is the sliding hernia, in which there is upward displacement of the esophagogastric junction and a portion of the proximal part of the stomach is herniated through the esophageal hiatus into the posterior mediastinum. Endoscopically, hiatal hernia is diagnosed when the mucosal esophagogastric junction is found more than 2 cm above the diaphragmatic hiatus impression. The diaphragmatic hiatus impression is usually located 40 cm from the incisor teeth, and the endoscopist identifies it by having the patient sniff or cough (see Plate 5). The presence of hiatal hernia should be carefully confirmed both during insertion and withdrawal of the instrument. With a large hernia, the herniated pouch can be readily seen moving up and down through the diaphragmatic hiatus during respiration. Prolapsed gastric mucosa may also be observed during the examination of some hiatal hernia patients who retch or gag.

Another technique to identify a hiatal hernia is to view the cardia from the gastric side by an intragastric **U** turn or **J** turn maneuver. The cardiac opening normally envelops the endoscope snugly as it exits through the cardia. If a sliding hiatal hernia is present, the opening forms an oval configuration around the instrument.

Esophagitis and Stricture

Within the normal esophageal mucosal surface is a network of fine red vessels. The early endoscopic recognition of esophagitis can be made when this vascular network is missing. When edema, erythema, nodularity, friability, erosions, and ulcerations appear, depending on the degree of inflammation, the diagnosis of esophagitis is readily established. Chronic reflux esophagitis is usually found at the distal esophagus in association with a herniated stomach; stricture formation develops at this level (see Plates 6 through 10). Esophageal moniliasis can be differentiated from reflux esophagitis by a white membrane scattered over most of the esophagus. When the plaque is pulled away, the underlying surface oozes blood (see Plate 11).

Esophageal Diverticula

Diverticula of the esophagus are thought to be acquired lesions that result from either the protrusion of mucosa through a defect in the esophageal musculature (pulsion diverticula), or from the traction effect of adjacent inflamed parabronchial lymphnodes (traction diverticula). There are three kinds of diverticula: (1) pharyngoesophageal pulsion diverticulum (Zenker's), (2) traction parabronchial or midesophageal diverticulum, and (3) pulsion epiphrenic diverticulum. These diverticula are readily demonstrated radiologically. Blind intubation of the esophagus in the presence of a pharyngoesophageal diverticulum is

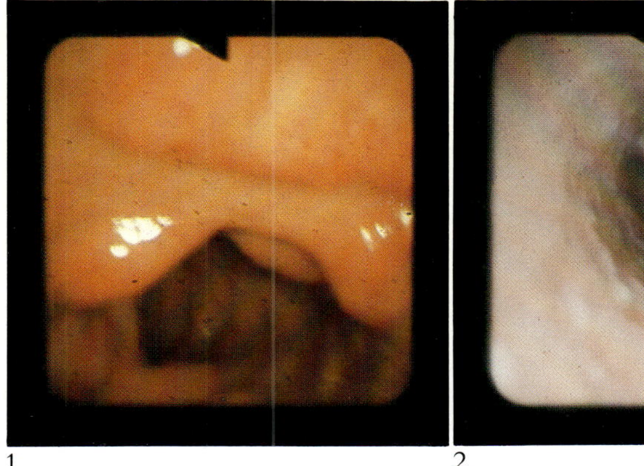

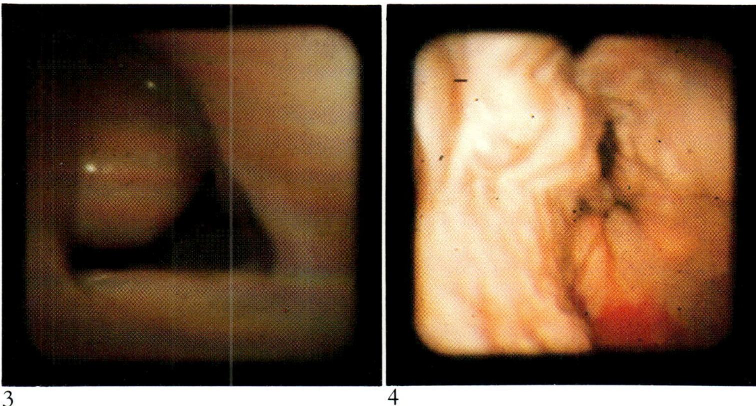

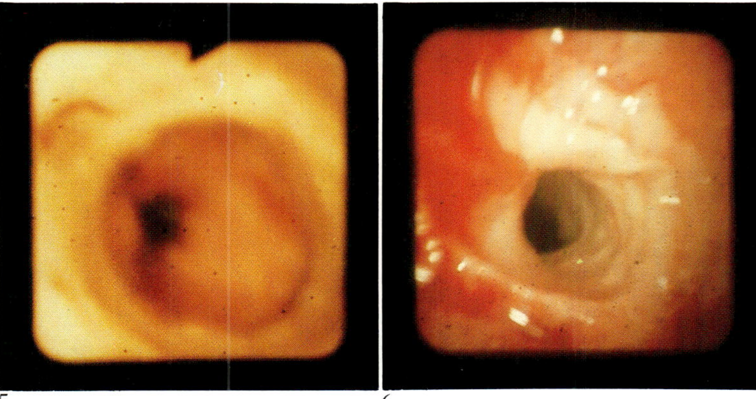

ESOPHAGUS

Plate 1.   Esophageal Cancer. This 53-year-old man had dysphagia for several weeks, and an esophagram demonstrated a mass in the midesophagus. A nonhemorrhagic mass is evident at the top of the picture. Biopsies demonstrated squamous cell carcinoma of the esophagus. If examination is delayed (as it frequently is in this disease), the cancer may narrow the lumen by encroaching submucosally, making a positive tissue diagnosis difficult to obtain.

Plate 2.   Esophageal Cancer. This shows a rather unusual presentation of squamous cell carcinoma of the esophagus. Ordinarily the cancer is diffuse and hemorrhagic, and only rarely presents in this polypoid fashion.

Plate 3.   Polyp. A large polyp is evident, partially blocking the lumen of the esophagus of a 56-year-old man who had increasing dysphagia for one and one-half years. This polyp has the appearance of a benign tumor, which is unusual in the esophagus and generally proves to be a submucosal leiomyoma. Because these lesions are covered by normal mucosa, endoscopic biopsies fail to demonstrate their true nature.

Plate 4.   Esophageal Varices. Varices are readily identified in the esophagus by their serpiginous longitudinal course extending from the distal esophagus as far as the cervical esophagus. The overlying mucosa is usually unchanged in color, but large distended varices which thin out the mucosa may give a bluish discoloration. If the question is whether esophageal varices are bleeding or not, as in this 44-year-old alcoholic woman, only esophagoscopy will provide the answer. In this photograph, fresh blood can be seen below the distended varix.

Plate 5.   Hiatal Hernia. This 55-year-old man had longstanding heartburn. The photograph shows esophagitis above the herniated stomach. Note the indentation of the diaphragm on the stomach.

Plate 6.   Hemorrhagic Esophagitis. This photograph shows marked hemorrhagic esophagitis with stricture formation. This disease occurred in a 68-year-old man who had persistent heartburn, and was found to be anemic. Biopsy confirmed the presence of esophagitis and made the possibility of concurrent esophageal cancer unlikely.

Plate 7. Following appropriate medical therapy and esophageal dilation, a good response to treatment of the problem presented in Plate 6 is shown.

Plate 8. Benign Stricture. A 71-year-old woman who had dysphagia for several years was found to have marked narrowing of the middle third of the esophagus with proximal dilation. The photograph demonstrates a severe stricture which by palpation with the endoscope and biopsy forceps suggested considerable cicatricial alteration. Biopsies of the mucosa above the stricture and brush cytology within the stricture did not identify malignant alteration. Dilation was carried out, utilizing the esophagoscope, by passing a wire with an obturator tip under direct vision through the area of stricture into the stomach. The stricture was then successfully dilated over a period of time, using the Eder-Puestow metal dilators.

Plate 9. Esophageal Ulcer. A prominent ulcer of the distal esophagus is obvious in this picture. A day before esophagoscopy, the patient had hematemesis and melena. This 59-year-old man had been under treatment for metastatic liposarcoma that was considered responsible for his severe retrosternal pain. Biopsies and brush cytology of the border of this ulcer failed to identify neoplastic infiltration. Esophageal ulceration ordinarily causes severe pain and frequently leads to massive hemorrhage. A chronic ulcer will penetrate the muscularis mucosae and lead to a marked fibrous reaction with stricture formation. Because of the marked inflammatory response and narrowing, barium examination of the esophagus may not lead to the identification of these ulcers, which are ordinarily diagnosed by esophagoscopy.

Plate 10. Schatzki Ring. A Schatzki ring that has just been dilated by the endoscope is shown. Blood is trickling from the edge of the ring, which has been split at that point. The ring is present at the esophagogastric junction and is not an uncommon occurrence, although the ring rarely narrows to 12 mm or less, the diameter at which dysphagia will occur. The ring in this 47-year-old patient caused infrequent episodes of dysphagia for 15 years but did not require dilation until the last 2 years.

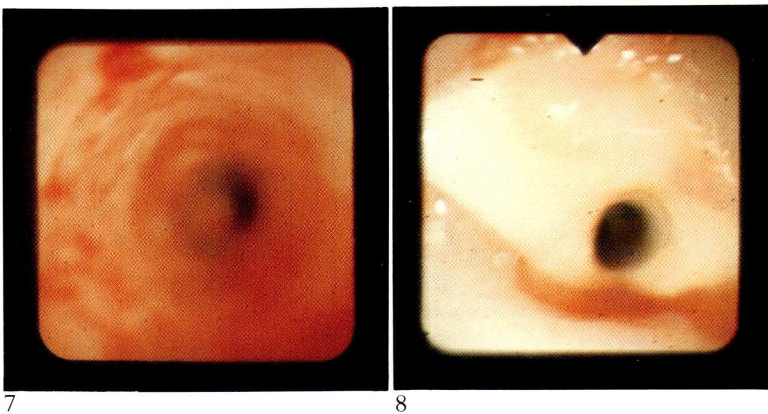

7 8

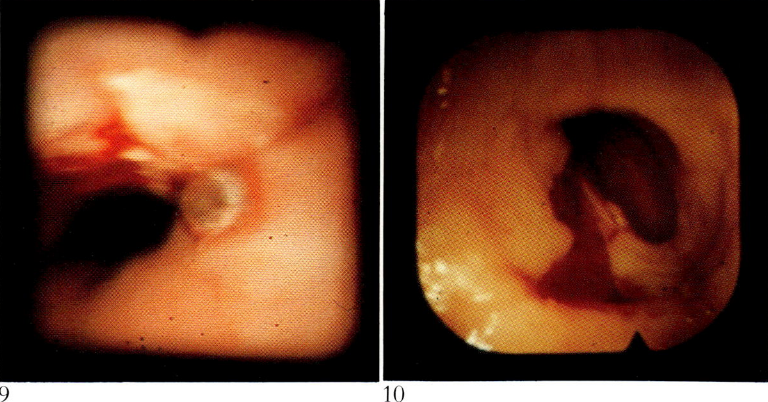

9 10

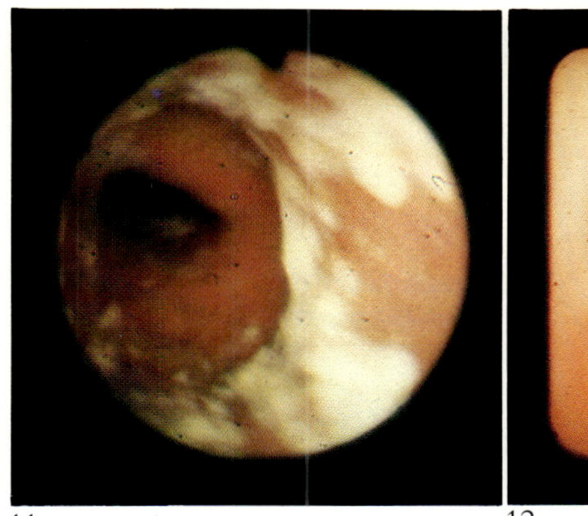
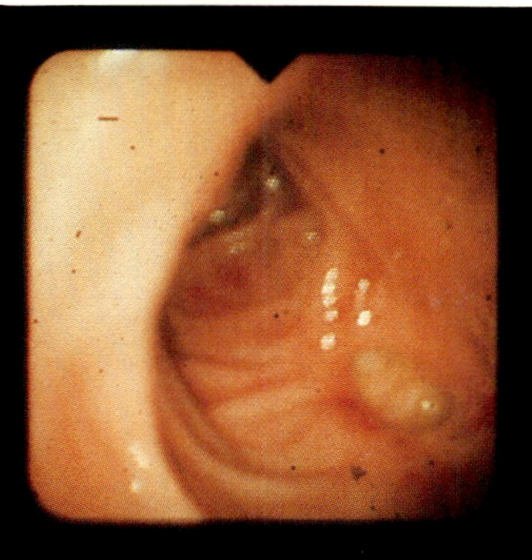

11   12

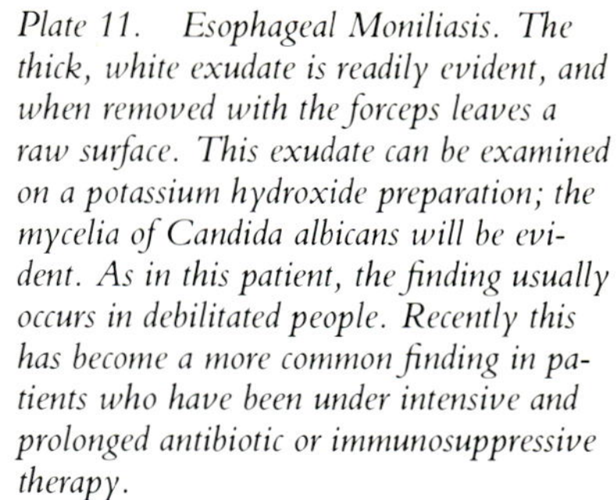

Plate 11.   Esophageal Moniliasis. The thick, white exudate is readily evident, and when removed with the forceps leaves a raw surface. This exudate can be examined on a potassium hydroxide preparation; the mycelia of Candida albicans will be evident. As in this patient, the finding usually occurs in debilitated people. Recently this has become a more common finding in patients who have been under intensive and prolonged antibiotic or immunosuppressive therapy.

Plate 12.   Diverticulum. The normal esophagus has a uniform appearance throughout its length. The mucosa varies from a pearl gray to a pale pink, and the surface is smooth and shiny. Folds are not found when the esophageal lumen is completely distended, but peristaltic waves may be evident. This photo shows the presence of a diverticulum of little clinical significance. There is some traction on the esophagus from this diverticulum, as evidenced by the radiating folds in contrast to the usual longitudinal folds seen when the esophagus is partially deflated.

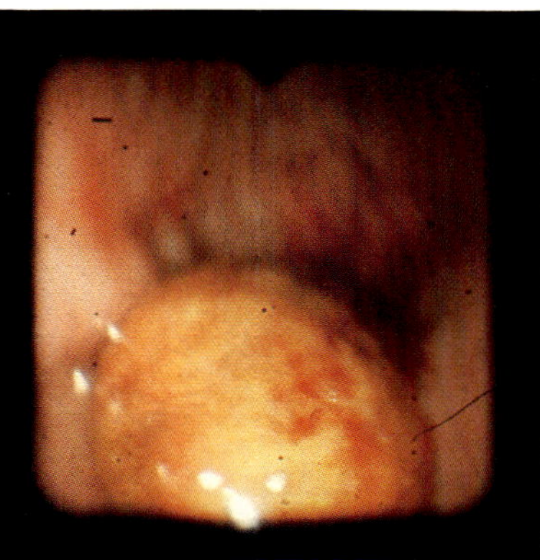

13

Plate 13.   Foreign Bodies. Foreign bodies can be successfully retrieved with fiberoptic endoscopes. Pictured here is a large nut that became impacted in the distal esophagus of a 50-year-old man while excitedly watching a televised football game. This nut was retrieved by snaring it with a wire loop used for polypectomies. Almost invariably there will be underlying pathology such as esophagitis, Schatzki ring, or cancer when food impaction occurs in the esophagus.

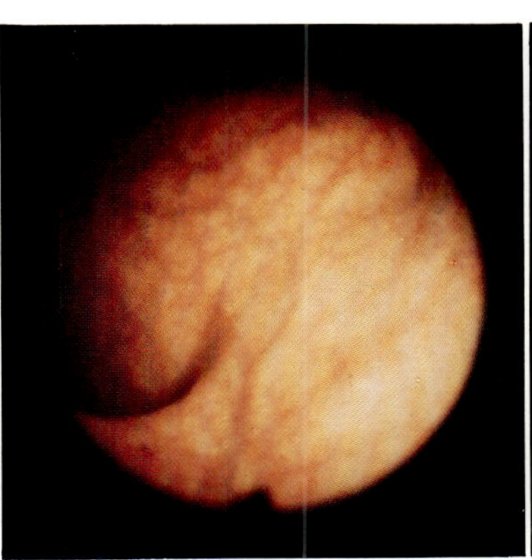
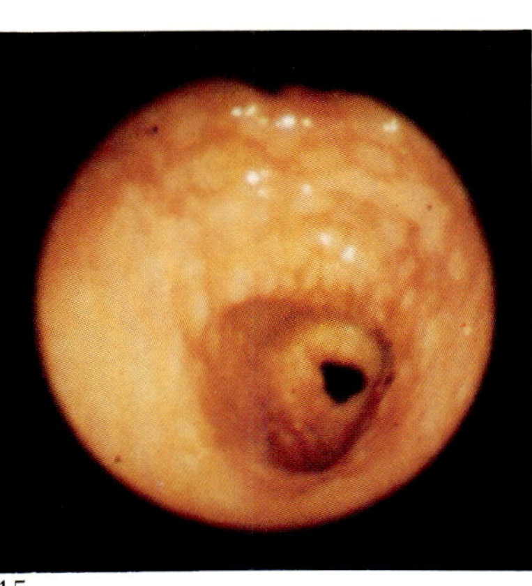

14   15

STOMACH

Plate 14.   Mucosal Atrophy. This photograph shows discoloration of the anterior wall proximal to the angulus. Blood vessels are clearly visible in the lower portion of the picture.

Plate 15.   Nodular Hyperplasia. Multiple hyperplastic nodules are seen in the antrum, especially on the anterior wall in association with atrophic gastritis.

Plate 16.   AGML. Multiple red erosions are seen on the greater curvature of the proximal stomach. This 35-year-old man had vomited blood after drinking a pint of vodka.

Plate 17.   AGML. Multiple black erosions are obvious in the antrum. Some of the erosions are red with central blackening. This 50-year-old man had taken aspirin for abdominal pain and proceeded to have hematemesis and melena.

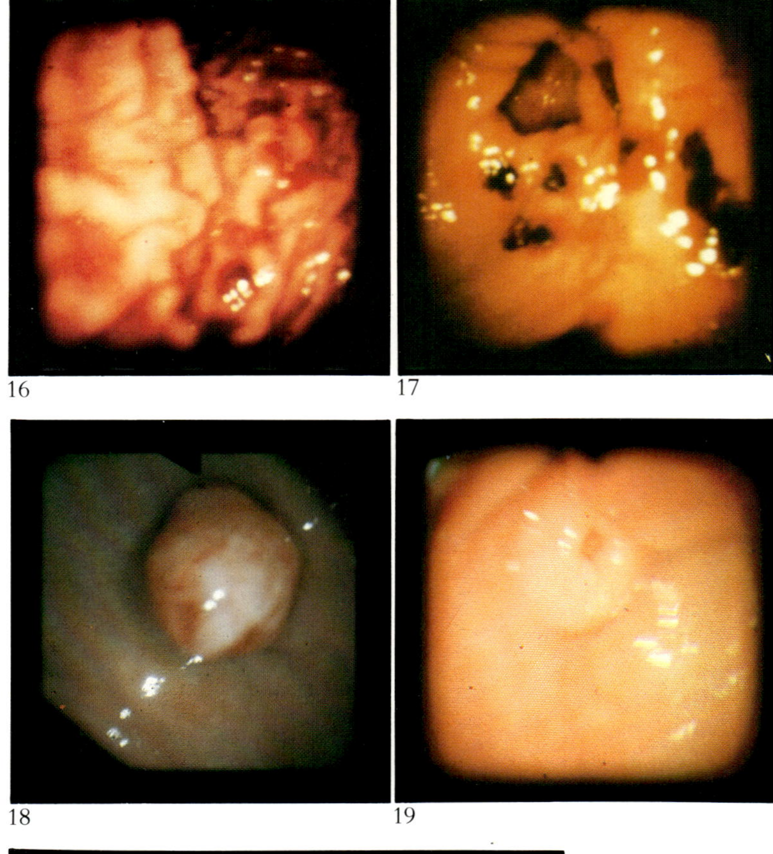

16   17

Plate 18.   Adenomatous Polyp. A benign polyp is seen on the lesser curvature of the gastric body. The polyp had a short stalk and polypectomy was successfully performed.

Plate 19.   Aberrant Pancreas. A submucosal tumor at the distal antrum is seen. The smooth surface is identical to the surrounding mucosa. A typical central dimple is present.

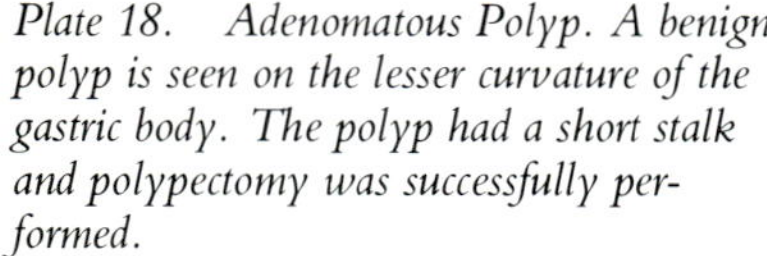

18   19

Plate 20.   Menetrier's Disease. This example of Menetrier's disease was diagnosed in a 56-year-old woman with marked hypoproteinemia. Multiple polypoid lesions hang from the anterior wall. Thick tortuous folds are noted on the greater curvature.

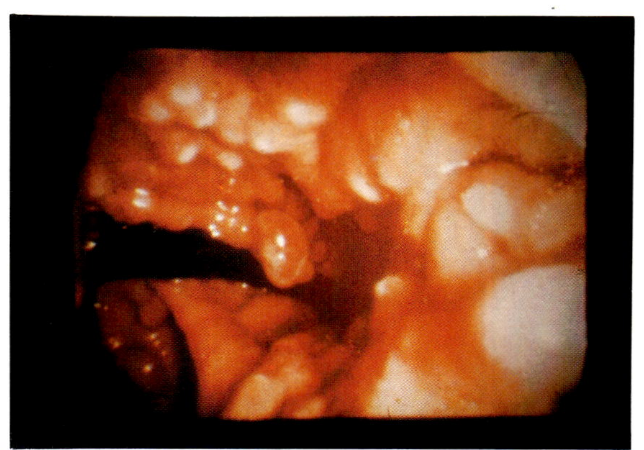

20

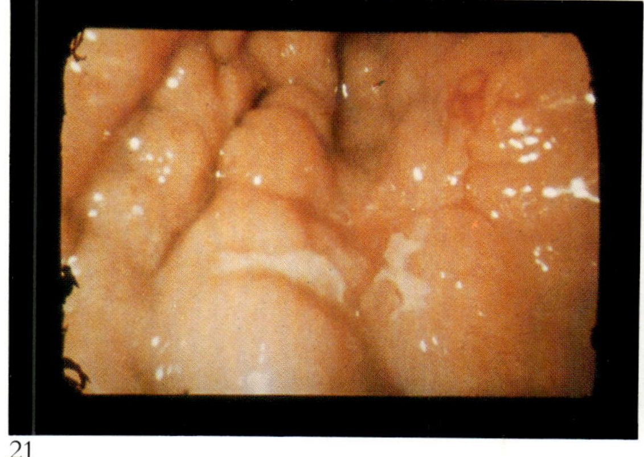

21

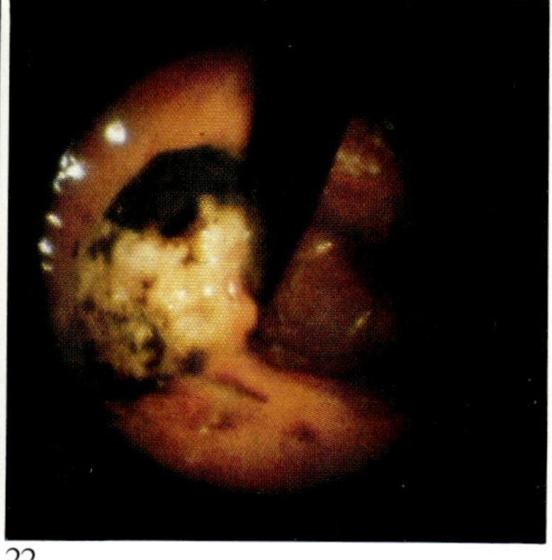

22

Plate 21.   Linitis Plastica. A carcinoma of Borrmann Type IV (linitis plastica) is shown here. Giant folds are noted on the greater curvature with irregular ulcerations. Biopsy of the margin of this ulcerated area showed malignant cells. When giant folds are found, adequate gastric distention is mandatory to find an ulcer.

Plate 22.   Benign Gastric Ulcer. An active benign ulcer on the lesser curvature of the lower body is shown. This deep ulcer has an undermined margin and fresh blood on the base. The picture was taken following a J-turn maneuver of the Olympus GIF type P2 gastroscope.

Plate 23.   Benign Gastric Ulcer. Another active ulcer is seen on the lesser curvature of the incisura. The ulcer base is white and deep, with a sharply demarcated margin.

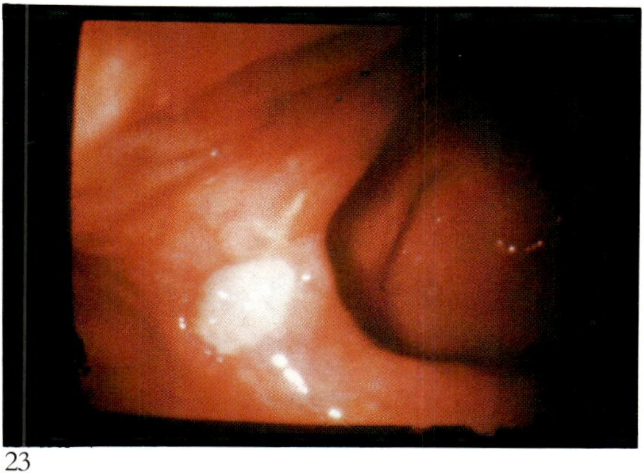

23

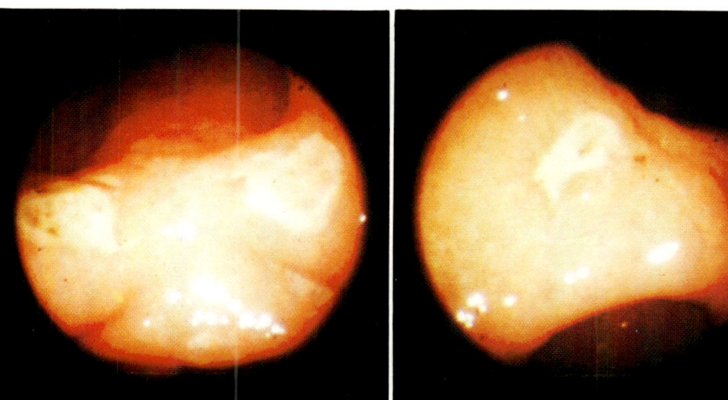

24   25

Plate 24.   Kissing Ulcers. Two ulcers are seen on the opposing walls of the lower body of the stomach that had an hour glass deformity.

Plate 25.   Healing Gastric Ulcer. An ulcer in the healing stage is seen on the lesser curvature of lower body. Note a narrow zone of reddening suggesting regenerating mucosa.

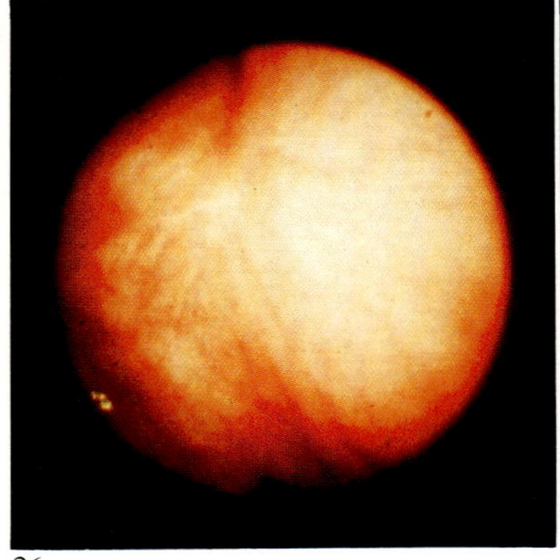
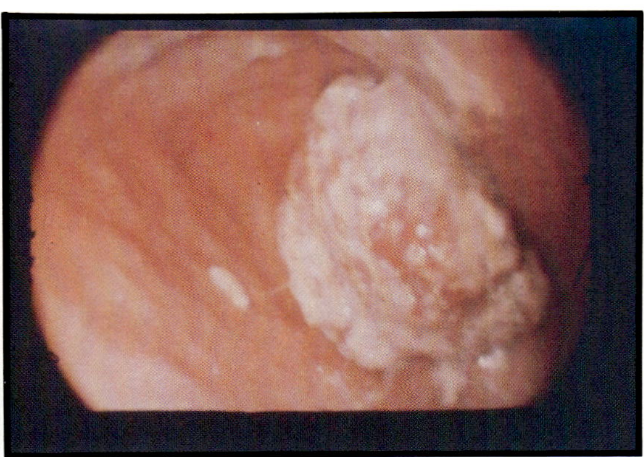

26   27

Plate 26.   Healed Gastric Ulcer. This ulcer, seen on the lesser curvature of the body of the stomach, is almost healed. Note the multiple converging mucosal folds from the posterior wall. The small white linear ulcer is still evident in the center of converging folds.

Plate 27.   Polypoid Carcinoma. A polypoid carcinoma of Borrmann Type I with broad base and irregular surface is seen on the midportion of the incisura.

Plate 28.   Ulcerating Carcinoma. A Borrmann Type III cancer is seen on the midportion of the incisura. Note that the proximal edge is destroyed.

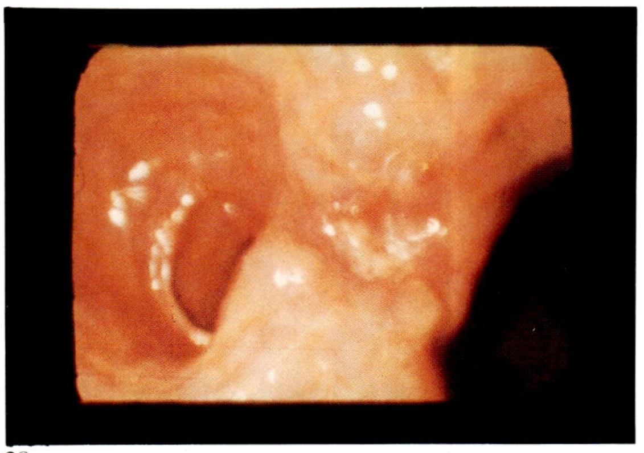

28

Plate 29.   Early Gastric Cancer. Type II C (superficial depressed type) early gastric cancer is seen on the posterior wall at the incisura. Note an irregular white depression with an island of mucosa. Converging mucosal folds show abrupt interruption.

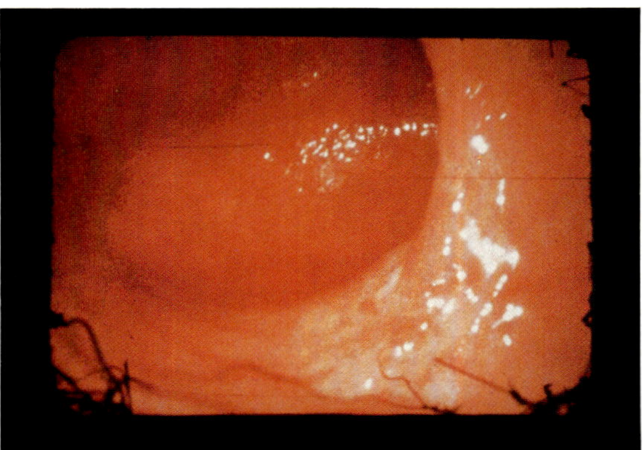

29

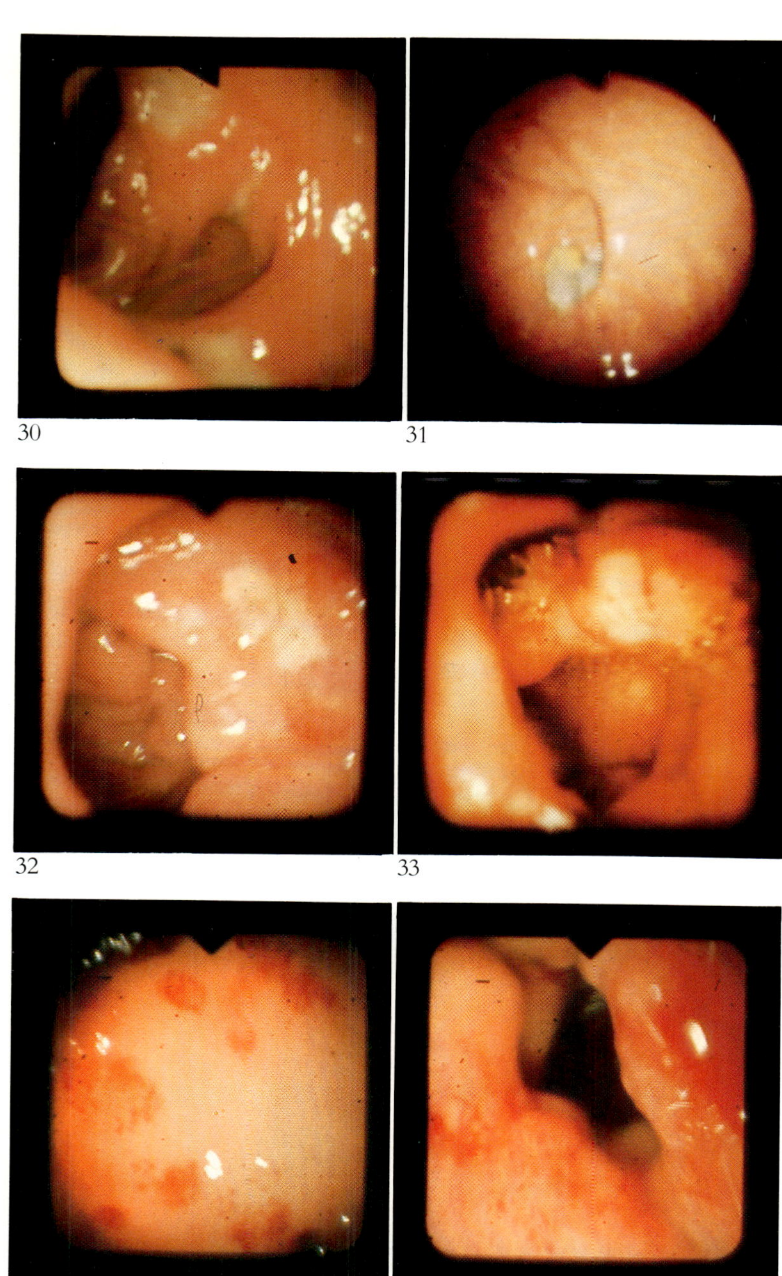

30

31

32

33

34

35

Plate 30.   Stomal Ulcer. Two white stomal ulcers are seen. One is at the gastric side of the anastomosis, and the other is at the junction of the afferent and efferent loops (a "jet" ulcer).

Plate 31.   Gastric Diverticulum. A diverticulum of the posterior wall near the cardia is shown, with its base of normal-appearing mucosa partially covered by mucus.

DUODENUM

Plate 32.   Duodenal Ulcer. This shows a superficial duodenal ulcer in the bulb. There is some thickening of the folds, suggesting associated edematous reaction.

Plate 33.   Duodenal Ulcer. In this deformed duodenal bulb, the ulcer could be visualized only briefly as the endoscope was withdrawn.

Plate 34.   Duodenitis. This shows multiple hemorrhagic areas in the duodenal bulb consistent with acute duodenitis. This finding occurred in a patient who had upper gastrointestinal bleeding, and at gastroscopy not only diffuse erosive gastritis predominantly in the antrum was identified, but also acute duodenitis. No specific ulcer was found either in the stomach or the duodenum.

Plate 35.   Duodenitis. This 49-year-old alcoholic patient had persistent nausea and vomiting. Upper gastrointestinal series demonstrated narrowing of the second portion of the duodenum, and the photograph confirms narrowing of the lumen of the descending duodenum with associated mucosal inflammatory reaction.

Plate 36.   Polyp. A large duodenal polyp is present just beyond the superior angle of the duodenum as indicated.

Plate 37.   Polyp from Plate 36. This shows the duodenal wall following duodenoscopic snare polypectomy. The polyp proved to be adenomatous in nature.

Plate 38.   Villous Adenoma. This 51-year-old patient was seen because of non-specific upper gastrointestinal symptoms and low-grade anemia. Upper gastro-intestinal series demonstrated a mass in the second portion of the duodenum. At duodenoscopy a friable mass in the mid-descending duodenum was revealed. Biop-sies were consistent with villous adenoma. Typical transverse folds of the descending duodenum are evident.

Plate 39.   Duodenal Cancer. This 49-year-old woman complained of vomiting and epigastric discomfort for six months. The upper gastrointestinal series showed a markedly irregular duodenal wall in the second portion. Gastroduodenoscopy re-vealed a hemorrhagic mass consistent with carcinoma of the duodenum, although biopsies and brush cytology failed to con-firm the impression. Biopsy of the mass at surgery demonstrated carcinoma of the duodenum. Metastases were present.

Plate 40.   Telangiectasias. This shows multiple telangiectasias within the duo-denum of a 74-year-old woman who had had recurrent upper gastrointestinal bleeding, unexplained by routine studies.

Plate 41.   Duodenal Diverticulum. This illustrates the normal mucosal appearance of the duodenum. This photograph was taken through the Olympus P2 pediatric panendoscope. The lumen of the duodenum is seen at the 6 o'clock position; at the 12 o'clock position, a diverticulum filled with debris is evident.

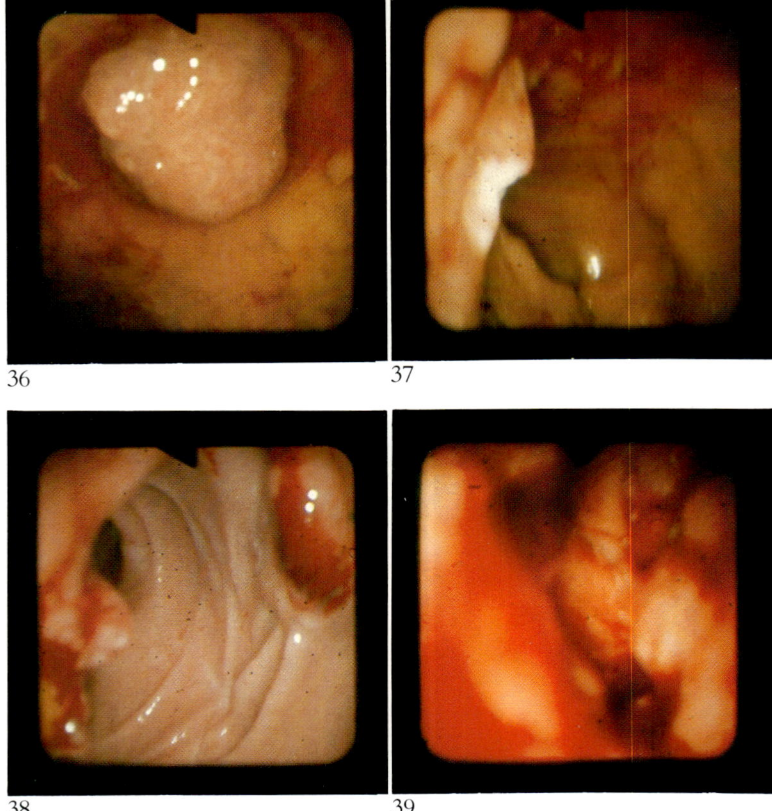

36   37

38   39

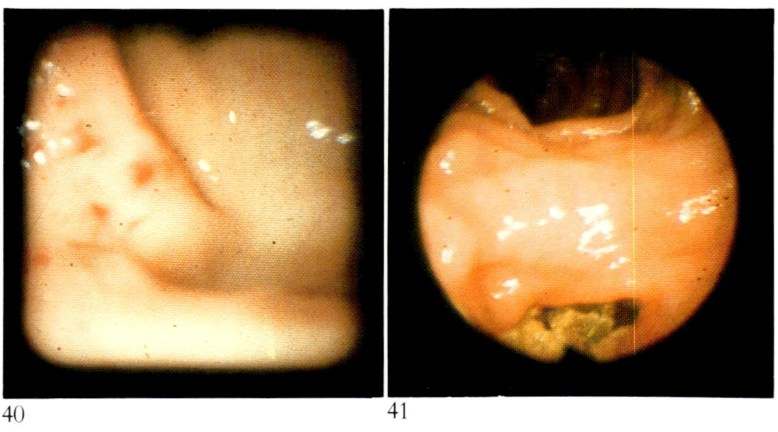

40   41

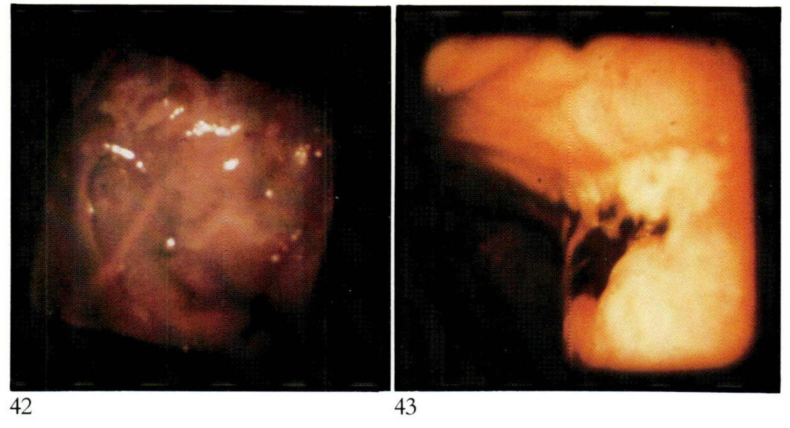

42

43

UPPER GI BLEEDING

Plate 42.   Blood from a varix spurts across the esophageal lumen.

Plate 43.   A Mallory-Weiss tear on the gastric side of the esophagogastric junction is filled with clotted blood.

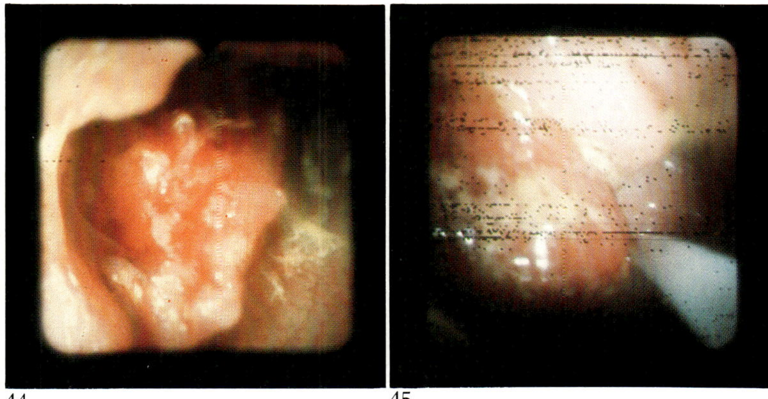

44

45

COLON

Plate 44.   This shows a polypoid mass in the middescending colon of an elderly lady who presented with unexplained anemia. The normal circular folds and pink mucosa of the colon are evident. This lesion was biopsied, and proved to be a villous adenoma.

Plate 45.   This is a photograph of a polyp at the hepatic flexure of the colon present in a 4-year-old patient. This child had episodes of bleeding and intussusception for 6 months. The polyp was removed with the patient under general anesthesia. The photograph shows the catheter containing the polypectomy snare.

Plate 46.   This is a photograph of the excised polyp, which proved to be juvenile in type.

Plate 47.   A 40-year-old executive who had a routine barium enema was found to have a 4-cm polyp in the cecum. This polyp was identified at colonoscopy, and electrocoagulation snare polypectomy was carried out. A diagnosis of cecal lipoma was made.

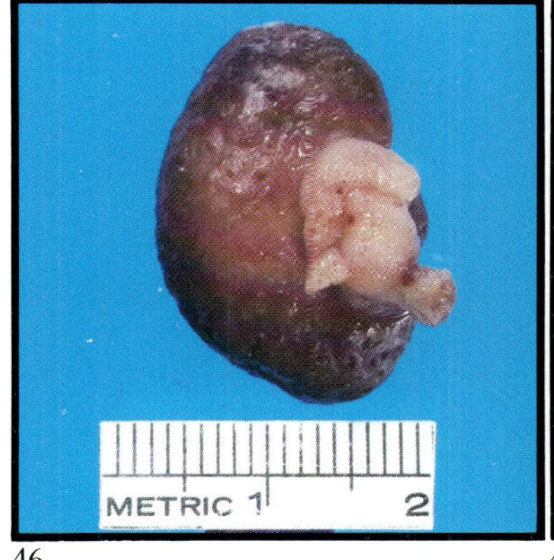

46

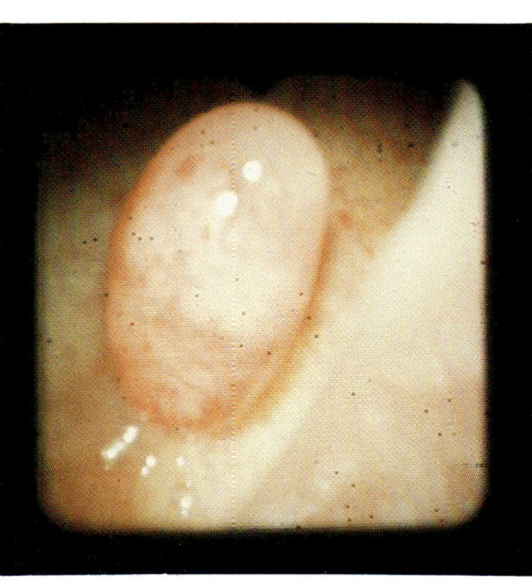

47

Plate 48. These are changes of chronic ulcerative colitis in a patient who has been on long-term corticosteroids. Inflammatory polypoid changes are evident although acute erosive manifestations are minimal.

Plate 49. A small red protuberance is seen projecting into the lumen at the level of the proximal sigmoid colon. This polyp was totally removed, and carcinoma in situ was identified pathologically. No further therapy was considered necessary.

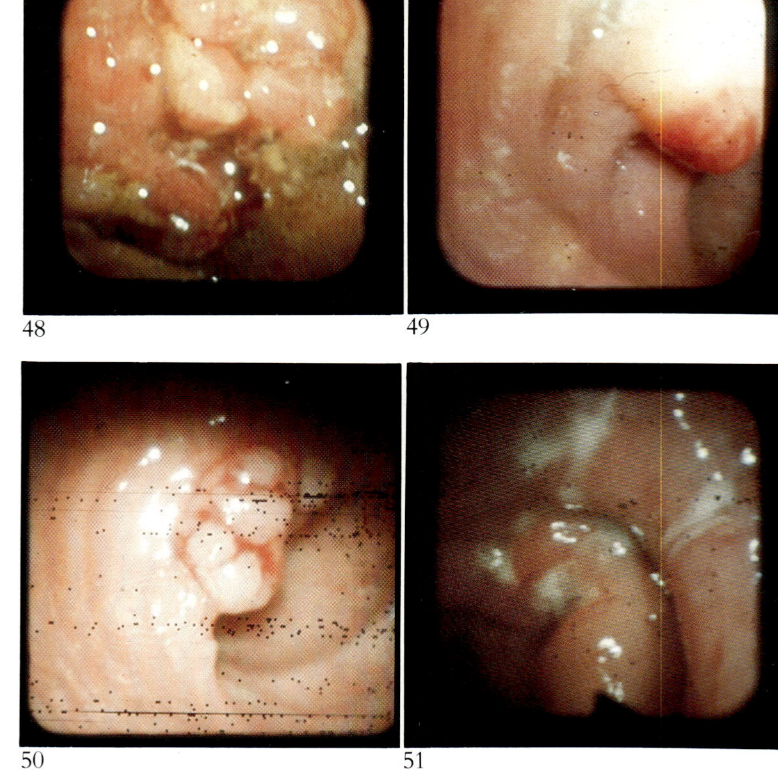

48
49

Plate 50. This shows a large hemorrhagic lesion characteristic of carcinoma of the colon which was proven by biopsy.

Plate 51. This 23-year-old woman had persistent diarrhea for several weeks. There was no blood in the stool. Sigmoidoscopic examination and barium enema study were not diagnostic. The colonoscopic findings are those of edematous folds of the descending colon with broad linear white-based ulcerations. This picture is consistent with granulomatous colitis although the biopsy of the lesion failed to demonstrate granuloma in the setting of acute inflammation.

50
51

Plate 52. This shows the biopsy forceps in place. The area of mucosa in the splenic flexure is hemorrhagic with multiple erosions. This young man had hematochezia unexplained by sigmoidoscopy and barium enema. The endoscopic and biopsy findings were consistent with acute ulcerative colitis.

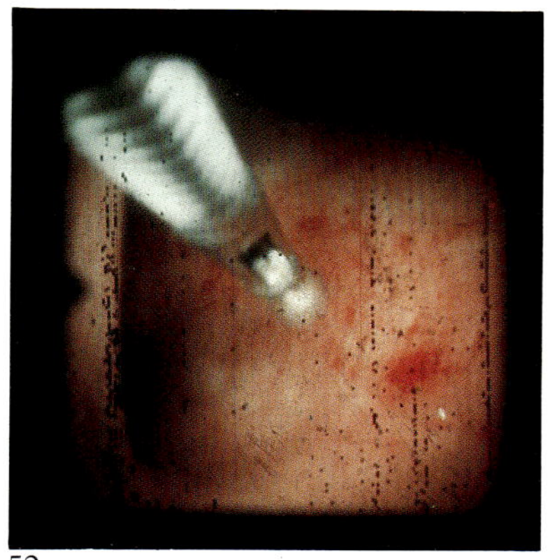

52

THERAPEUTIC ENDOSCOPY

Plate 53. The needle is seen in the duodenal bulb prior to removal by means of forceps.

Plate 54. Juvenile polyp in the descending colon of a 3-year-old child. The polypectomy snare is being placed about the pedicle.

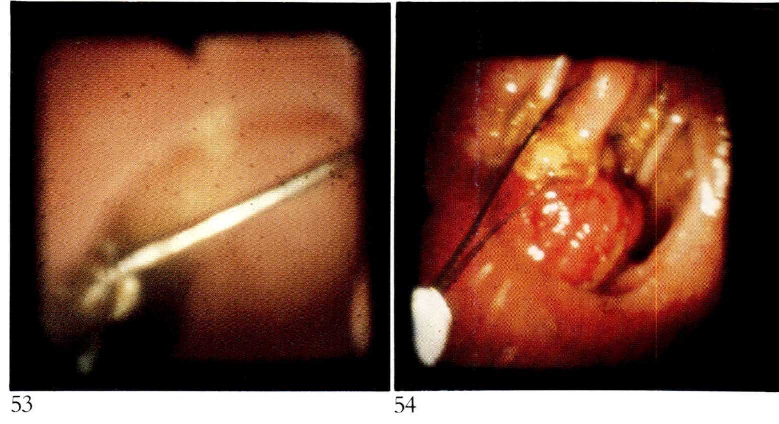

53
54

dangerous; direct vision is always recommended if no upper gastrointestinal series has been done before endoscopy.

A diverticulum appears endoscopically as a smooth, round opening or mucosal depression (see Plate 12). Small diverticula as well as those with a narrow neck are easily missed by endoscopy, which is not really required to establish the diagnosis of diverticulum but should be performed to identify associated esophagitis.

Motility Disorders

Esophageal motility disorders such as achalasia, hypotensive lower esophageal sphincter, or diffuse esophageal spasm are diagnosed by radiologic and manometric study. Endoscopy is required to differentiate between achalasia and either benign stricture or carcinoma of the distal esophagus. Achalasia is confirmed when endoscopy demonstrates a tight sphincter with a rosette pattern of converging esophageal folds. Retained secretions, food particles, and esophagitis are often found (see Plate 13). The endoscope can be inserted through the tight sphincter by firm pressure. It is important to see the cardia (using a retroflexion maneuver) to rule out cardiac cancer.

STOMACH

Diffuse Gastric Mucosal Lesions

Superficial gastritis cannot be diagnosed dependably by endoscopy or roentgenographic examination; it requires a biopsy for accurate diagnosis. Endoscopic biopsy provides a correct diagnosis in most instances, and multiple biopsies can determine the exact extent of the gastritis. There are two types of diffuse mucosal lesions: gastric atrophy and acute gastric mucosal lesions or erosive gastritis; they can be consistently diagnosed by their endoscopic appearance.

GASTRIC ATROPHY. Endoscopically, gastric mucosal atrophy presents as a thin, transparent, pallid, grayish mucosa through which an underlying submucosal vascular pattern is readily visible (see Plate 14). The term *gastric atrophy* is appropriate for gastroscopy, rather than atrophic gastritis, since any inflammatory component can only be proven by histologic examination. Mucosal atrophy is often associated with achlorhydria, and is always found in pernicious anemia. Atrophic gastritis may be accompanied by hyperplastic nodules or polyps (see Plate 15).

ACUTE GASTRIC MUCOSAL LESIONS. Acute gastric mucosal lesions (AGML) are characterized by multiple superficial mucosal lesions most often diagnosed by endoscopy when bleeding occurs. Terms such as *acute erosive gastritis, acute hemorrhagic gastritis, stress ulcer, Cushing's ulcer,* and *Curling's ulcer* are encompassed by AGML. Some lesions may penetrate deeper than the muscularis mucosae histologically and are, in fact, ulcers rather than erosions. Since the causes of these lesions are multiple and some of the lesions are acute ulcers, the term *acute gastric mucosal lesion* seems more appropriate to describe this phenomenon that may bring about serious mucosal bleeding.

Endoscopic changes in AGML include petechiae, red erosions, black erosions, red erosions with central blackening, and white-based erosions; these are all the same lesion at different stages of development (see Plates 16 and 17).

The mucosal lesions caused by stress gastritis due to trauma or sepsis usually occur in the proximal half of the stomach, and spread to the distal stomach with increasing severity. Mucosal lesions caused by alcohol consist, for the most part, of red–based erosions that are usually located in the proximal half of the stomach. Aspirin erosions occur distally; some have a deep white base. The healing processes of mucosal erosions are identical in the three groups. As observed endoscopically, two distinct patterns that depend on the degree of mucosal change can be noted. In more severe cases, the progression from red–based erosions to complete healing goes through stages of blackening of the base, marginal swelling, white fibrinous change, and finally of a light red covering of regenerating mucosa. In milder cases, red–based erosions become gradually less red, and blend into the surrounding mucosa without passing through the successive changes of the severe group.

A nasogastric suction tube may cause mucosal hemorrhage, petechiae, and erosions that are found on the greater curvature side of the stomach in a linear distribution.

Polypoid Lesions of the Stomach
A gastric polyp may be adenomatous or may simply represent mucosal hyperplasia. Mucosal elevation due to submucosal tumor such as aberrant pancreas or leiomyoma is not, strictly speaking, a polyp; it is better described as a protruding lesion. It can be difficult to differentiate a polyp from a submucosal tumor endoscopically.

Yamada described four categories of gastric protruding lesions, including polyps as well as submucosal tumors (see Fig. 4–1):

Type I is a flat, smooth lesion without a definite border.

Type II is a flat lesion with a definite border sloping from the normal mucosa without indentation.

Type III is a protruded lesion with a definite indentation at the mucosal margin without a stalk.

Type IV is a pedunculate polyp with a distinct stalk.

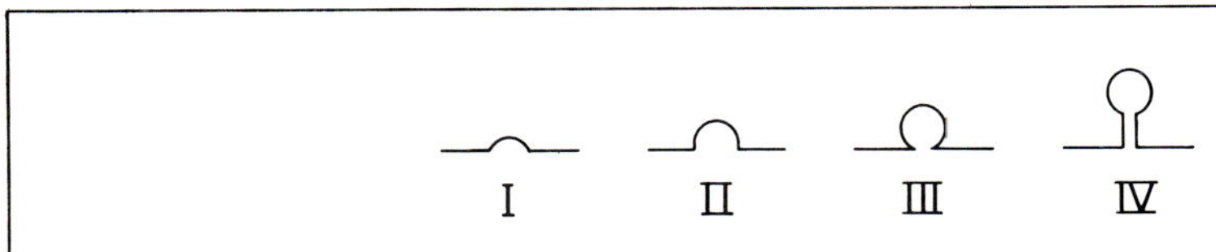

Figure 4-1.   The four types of gastric protruding lesions (Yamada's classification).

There is a definite relationship between the type of protrusion and the histologic finding. For example, a certain form of early gastric cancer belongs in the Type II polyp category, and a Borrmann Type I polypoid cancer is usually a Type III polypoid lesion. Submucosal tumors are, for the most part, Type I in character. Smooth, round, pedunculate polyps less than 2 cm in diameter are almost always benign adenomas (see Plate 18).

Benign submucosal tumors include leiomyoma, fibroma, lipoma, neurofibroma, and aberrant pancreas. In general, submucosal tumors are hemispheric, with a broad base showing gradual transition into the surrounding mucosa. Occasionally one or more mucosal folds stretch from the surrounding mucosa over the surface of the tumor as bridging folds. Aberrant pancreas is usually located in the antrum; the polyp can be readily recognized by its central dimple (see Plate 19).

The biopsy technique depends on the type and size of the protruding lesion. The mucosa overlying the submucosal tumor can be lifted off by the biopsy forceps, but this will not provide a positive diagnosis for the tumor itself. To obtain submucosal tissue, a large particle biopsy, hot biopsy, or a lift-and-cut biopsy employing a snare may be used. A polyp with a stalk is best removed in toto by snare polypectomy.

Giant Gastric Folds

Prominent folds along the greater curvature of the stomach are frequently recognized in the course of upper gastrointestinal series. These folds can generally be effaced by compression but when this does not occur, the possibility of an underlying abnormality must be considered. The borderline between normal large folds and *giant gastric folds* is hazy, and frequently only gastroscopic evaluation and biopsy will settle the issue. Gastroscopic examination defines folds as giant when they appear broad, tortuous, and at times, even polypoid in nature. Distention of the stomach with air does not flatten this type of abnormal fold pattern. Ordinarily, giant folds occur in the area where prominent normal folds are seen, that is, along the greater curvature of the stomach; but giant folds may be seen in any segment of the stomach or may indeed involve the entire stomach.

The etiology of giant folds varies. At one end of the causal spectrum, giant folds may simply represent functional changes of the muscularis mucosae or engorgement of the mucosa and submucosa. At the other end, however, infiltrating or scirrhous carcinoma or lymphoma may be responsible for the formation of giant folds. Between the benign and malignant processes there are a number of rare disease entities that must be separated by gastroscopic biopsy.

The giant folds may be due primarily to mucosal thickening that can occur with nonspecific gastritis. In Ménétrier's disease, mucosal thickening is the result of hypertrophy of the muscularis mucosae in association with cystic glandular changes (see Plate 20). The gastroscopic appearance of the Zollinger-Ellison syndrome may be indistinguishable from that of Ménétrier's disease. In the former case, however, the giant folds are a result of glandular hyperplasia. Clinically, the two are readily separated by the presence of excessive hydrochloric acid in the Zollinger-Ellison syndrome and low acid output in Ménétrier's disease.

Giant folds may be related to submucosal infiltration. There is no way to distinguish endoscopically such conditions as sarcoidosis, tuberculosis, or Crohn's disease.

If a specific diagnosis is to be made, gastric biopsy will be necessary. Unfortunately, the usual gastroscopic forceps biopsy is inadequate for accurate histologic evaluation. A bigger biopsy can be obtained by using a large bayonet forceps (biopsy forceps with a central spike) through the biopsy channel, or the Carey suction biopsy capsule may be positioned in the stomach under endoscopic control in an area of giant fold. Unfortunately, submucosal disease such as lymphoma, sarcoidosis, or linitis plastica will usually not be identified by this technique (see Plate 21). A "jumbo" biopsy done with the polypectomy snare enhances the opportunity for a tissue diagnosis, but carries with it increased risk of bleeding or postbiopsy ulceration. A panendoscope with a large biopsy channel 3.7 mm in diameter is now available (Olympus GIF-IT), and large biopsy specimens can be safely obtained using large forceps with a central spike. Sometimes a definitive diagnosis can only be obtained by full-thickness biopsy at operation.

Gastric Ulcer

Endoscopically, typical benign gastric ulcers appear as sharply demarcated ulcerations with a gray-to-white base. The shape of the ulcer is usually round or oval (see Plates 22 and 23), but irregularly shaped ulcers can be found. Gastric ulcers penetrate the muscularis mucosae into the submucosa, and even the muscularis propria or serosa, whereas the erosion is only a mucosal defect. Most gastric ulcers are located along the lesser curvature and usually occur at the incisura angularis. Multiple ulcers can be found, and occasionally two ulcers are seen on opposing walls of the stomach ("kissing" ulcers, see Plate 24).

A deformity of the gastric wall induced by an ulcer is caused by the fibrotic contraction of healing. Henning's sign is a gothic-arch deformity caused by an ulcer or scar on the lesser curvature at the incisura. An hourglass configuration is caused by a thick fold running transversely through the anterior and posterior walls, overriding the greater curvature and frequently a result of "kissing" ulcers (Plate 24).

Endoscopically, ulcers can be found in any of four stages, according to the clinical course and histologic study.

ACTIVE ULCER STAGE.   The ulcer is round or oval, with the surrounding mucosa showing a marked swelling and occasionally diffuse reddening. While the overall ulcer margin is sharply demarcated, the ulcer bed frequently encroaches over a part of the margin as a result of exacerbation. The ulcer crater is often deep and undermined (Plates 22 and 23); sometimes there is an abrupt secondary excavation of the base. The base shows a thick white coating often speckled with brown or black. The convergence of mucosal folds is rarely noted in the acute stage.

REGRESSIVE STAGE.   The edematous swelling and diffuse erythema of the surrounding mucosa subside, virtually disappearing in the next, or healing stage. A narrow zone of reddening may also lend a velvety appearance; it surrounds a part of the ulcer edge (see Plate 25).

HEALING STAGE.   As the reddening gradually intensifies throughout the healing stage, a red halo forms around the ulcer.

The convergence of mucosal folds gradually becomes distinct in the regressive and healing stage. The surrounding mucosa is less elevated. The clean white coating over the bottom of the ulcer develops a yellowish tone, and becomes thinner as the ulcer shrinks and heals (see Plate 26).

SCARRING STAGE.   The surface of the ulcer shows a depression with velvetlike reddening or a gray-yellow lackluster surface (Plate 26). No coating can be seen on it. While such reddening may be longlived, the scar usually loses its color as time passes. Around the scar, convergence of mucosal folds is usually evident.

Gastric Cancer

ADVANCED CANCER.   The endoscopic diagnosis of advanced gastric cancer that has extended beyond the submucosa is not difficult. The endoscopic appearance of an advanced cancer conforms to one of the four types of gastric cancer of Borrmann's classification.

Type I is a polypoid carcinoma characterized by localized protuberances of various size. This cancer has a broad base, and a biopsy specimen is readily obtained (see Plate 27).

Type II is a noninfiltrating malignant ulcer, the edge of which is usually raised and nodular, but limited sharply by surrounding mucosa. The mucosal folds converging on the tumor are interrupted before they reach the edge.

Type III is an infiltrative carcinomatous ulcer; the edge is partly destroyed by cancer (see Plate 28).

Type IV is a diffuse infiltrating carcinoma, and the gastric wall becomes rigid (linitis plastica). Some mucosal changes such as shallow or deep ulcerations (Plate 21) and nodular elevations may be seen. If there are no mucosal changes endoscopic diagnosis is difficult, and a deep biopsy will be required for diagnosis.

EARLY GASTRIC CARCINOMA.   Early gastric carcinoma is defined as carcinoma limited to the mucosa and submucosa, regardless of the size or the presence of lymphnode metastasis. There are three major types of early gastric cancer (see Fig. 4-2).

Type I is the protruded or polypoid type that is easily recognized through the gastroscope but is relatively rare.

Type II is a superficial cancer further subdivided into three categories: Type IIa (elevated), Type IIb (flat), and Type IIc (depressed). *Type IIa* has an elevation less than twice the thickness of the mucosa. The surface of the elevation is usually irregular with a central depression.

Figure 4-2.   The three types of early gastric cancer (From the classification proposed in 1962 by the Japan Gastroenterological Endoscopy Society)

Macroscopic Classification of Early Gastric Carcinoma

Type I   Protruded Type
   Protrusion into the gastric lumen is prominent.

Type II   Superficial Type
   Unevenness of the surface is not obvious.

   Type IIa   Elevated Type
      The surface is slightly elevated.
   Type IIb   Flat Type
      Almost no recognizable elevation or depression from the surrounding mucosa is present.
   Type IIc   Depressed Type
      The surface is slightly depressed.

Type III   Excavated Type
   An excavation in the gastric wall is prominent.

When the carcinoma shows diverse morphological patterns, 2 or more types are described together, e.g. type III + IIc or IIc + III. The first Roman numeral indicates the predominant pattern.

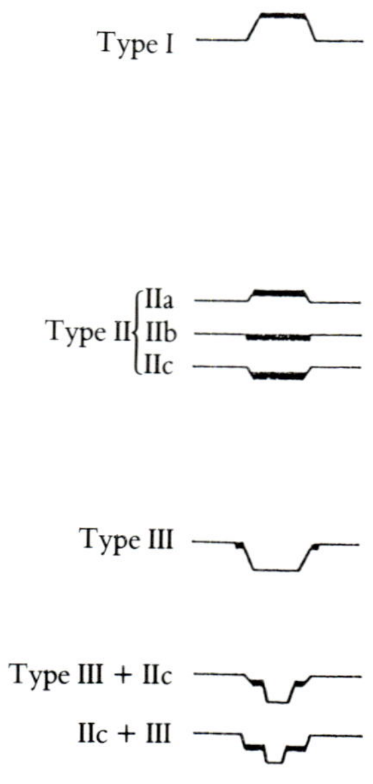

Type IIb is the most difficult to identify, but may be suspected on finding discoloration and surface dullness. *Type IIc* is the most common, and occasionally combines with other types. Type IIc shows an irregular white depression, occasionally with an island of mucosa inside (see Plate 29). Converging mucosal folds often show abrupt, moth-eaten interruption, and club-shaped thickening.

Type III is the excavated or ulcerated type, and is usually impossible to distinguish from a benign ulcer. The excavated area is frequently surrounded by a depressed zone (Type IIc), and the predominant pathology may be of either Type III or Type IIc.

To find early gastric cancer, the endoscopist must be suspicious of slight mucosal changes. Biopsy, touch smear, brush cytology, and close follow-up are mandatory.

In Japan, the incidence of gastric cancer is very high, and endoscopy or gastrocamera examination is widely used for screening purposes. About one third of all cancers in Japan are diagnosed in the early stage, so that a high five-year survival rate follows surgical treatment. In the United States, the incidence of gastric cancer is low, but nonetheless the American endoscopist should be prepared to recognize the early resectable stage.

Postoperative Stomach

STOMAL ULCER.   Patients with complaints after gastric surgery pose difficult diagnostic problems. These are the patients who have had gastrectomy with either gastroduodenostomy (Billroth I), gastrojejunostomy (Billroth II), or a pyloroplasty. Surgical distortion of the stomach by the creation of an anastomosis or pyloroplasty produces confusing niches and folds for the radiologist. Many recurrent or anastomotic ulcers escape detection, and false positive diagnoses are not unusual in radiologic study. Fiberoptic endoscopy allows a thorough investigation of the area and furnishes a definitive diagnosis.

The difficult areas for endoscopic examination after gastric surgery are the immediate jejunal side of a gastrojejunostomy or the immediate duodenal side of a gastroduodenostomy. The side-viewing and pediatric endoscopes are useful when there is a question of a lesion in those areas. Most ulcers are located at the stoma or in the small intestine within a few centimeters of the stoma. They are not commonly found in the stomach remnant. In a double-barreled stoma, a "jet" ulcer is not infrequently seen at the junction of the afferent and efferent loops (see Plate 30).

GASTRITIS.   Postoperative gastritis is commonly seen about the stoma, and does not cause symptoms other than those caused by gastritis in the intact stomach—a variable and undefinable symptom complex.

Diffuse hyperemia or radiating bands of hyperemia along the greater curvature of the stomach remnant can be seen in patients with a considerable amount of bile in the stomach. This bile reflux gastritis may occur with persistent abdominal pain and bilious vomiting. Patients whose biopsy specimens show marked inflammatory change may benefit from a surgical diversion of the bile.

CANCER.   In the majority of cases, the finding of cancer represents a tumor recurrence, and the endoscopic diagnosis is apparent. Pseudopolypoid formation at the anastomosis due to suture granulation may be differentiated from cancer with difficulty. Adenocarcinoma has recently been found in postoperative stomachs of 20 years (or more) duration. Annual endoscopic evaluation and biopsy of these old operated stomachs is recommended to detect early gastric cancer.

SUTURES.   Retained sutures of black silk are often seen in the area of anastomosis. These sutures are generally of no clinical significance, but occasionally cause ulceration and bleeding. The sutures are safely removed by suture-cutting forceps or by "hot" biopsy forceps passed through the endoscope.

Gastric Diverticulum

The gastric diverticulum is usually diagnosed by upper gastrointestinal series but occasionally may be misinterpreted as an ulcer. The diverticulum causes no symptoms (see Plate 31).

DUODENUM

Duodenal Ulcer

Duodenal ulcers occur in the duodenal bulb in a variety of shapes (see Plates 32 and 33). If the duodenal bulb is deformed from recurrent ulceration and scarring, careful examination will be necessary to find the crater. *Bulbar ulcers* are readily identified as 3-to-5 mm, round, superficial craters, but may reach a width of a few centimeters and be quite deep. *Channel ulcers* or ulcers in the fornices may be difficult to find. At times, both forward-viewing and lateral-viewing duodenoscopes are necessary to avoid overlooking a bulbar ulcer (see Plate 33).

Duodenitis

Duodenitis as an endoscopic diagnosis is subject to considerable controversy. Although the duodenal mucosa may appear erythematous and the folds prominent, there is usually poor histologic correlation for these findings. When actual erosions and hemorrhage occur, villous abnormalities and inflammatory infiltrate may then be found on microscopic examination. Whether this type of nonspecific duodenitis (localized primarily to the bulb) is related to the formation of a duodenal ulcer or represents an interim healing stage of a duodenal ulcer has been a matter of debate. *Peptic duodenitis* has been described in association with severe hemorrhage from the first portion of the duodenum (see Plate 34). These changes are also cited as being associated with acute and chronic alcoholism (see Plate 35), but the validity of this observation is no more certain with duodenitis than it is with gastritis. Even when there is a histologically identifiable lesion, it is exceedingly difficult to relate the pathologic change to any clinical state. Since this nonspecific duodenitis resembles that which occurs in association with duodenal ulcers, the possibility exists that the ulcer simply was not seen.

Specific diseases induce duodenitis. *Brunner's gland hyperplasia* may lead to coarse duodenal folds that, when biopsied, often show inflammatory changes or lymphoid hyperplasia. Brunner's gland hyperplasia is almost always revealed by endoscopic biopsy. At times, Brunner's gland hyperplasia may present as a polypoid mass; this can be removed by duodenoscopic polypectomy.

Lymphoid hyperplasia may induce mucosal irregularity of the duodenum. Duodenoscopic biopsy is usually successful in identifying this abnormality.

Crohn's disease of the duodenum may cause severe changes characterized by erythema, friability, edema, and thickening of the duodenal wall. Frequently associated ulcerations, unlike peptic ulcers, are irregular in contour. Because of the submucosal nature of this disease, mucosal biopsies usually fail to demonstrate the typical noncaseating granulomata.

Duodenal Neoplasms

The most common benign tumor encountered in the duodenum is the adenoma (see Plate 36). This may be of the typical tubular type or the tumor may show villous change (see Plate 38). When tumors arise from the submucosa, they are usually either lipomas or leiomyomas. These neoplasms are ordinarily found incidentally in the course of an upper gastrointestinal series, but may occasionally bleed and bring about bowel obstruction. When the adenoma or lipoma is pedunculate, duodenoscopic polypectomy may be done (see Plate 37). A number of successful cases have been reported.

Adenocarcinoma is first in incidence for cancer of the duodenum (see Plate 39). Carcinoid tumors, sarcomas, and lymphomas occur rarely. Carcinoma is frequently periampullary, or there may be a primary carcinoma of the papilla itself. Pancreatic cancer may invade the duodenal wall and appear as a primary cancer of the duodenum. Melanoma metastasizes to the duodenum as it does to the stomach.

Telangiectasias

Telangiectasias may be seen as part of Rendu-Osler-Weber Syndrome or may occur as an isolated phenomenon. At the time of bleeding, the underlying vascular anomaly may not be recognized. Following blood replacement and with a dry field the telangiectasias become obvious (see Plate 40).

Duodenal Diverticulum

Diverticula commonly develop in the second portion of the duodenum. The diverticulum is rarely the cause of symptoms. The papilla of Vater is found in close proximity to or even in the diverticulum (see Plate 41).

SELECTED READINGS

Belber, J.P. Gastroscopy and Duodenoscopy. In M.H. Sleisenger and J.S. Fordtran (eds.), *Gastrointestinal Disease*. Philadelphia: Saunders, 1978. Pp. 691–713.

Demling, L., Ottenjann, R., and Elster, K. *Endoscopy and Biopsy of the Esophagus and Stomach*. Translated by K.H. Soergel. Philadelphia: Saunders, 1972.

Hattori, K., Winans, C.S., and Archer, F. Endoscopic diagnosis of esophageal inflammation. *Gastrointest. Endosc.* 20:102, 1974.

Haubrich, W.S. Recent advances in gastrointestinal endoscopy: A critical evaluation. In *Developments in Digestive Disease*. Philadelphia: Lea & Febiger, 1977.

Katz, D., and Siegel, H.I. Erosive gastritis and acute gastrointestinal mucosal lesions. *Prog. Gastroenterol.* 1:67, 1968.

Martin, T.R., et al. Lift and cut biopsy technique for submucous sampling. *Gastrointest. Endosc.* 23:29, 1976.

Menguy, R. Gastritis and Gastric Ulcer. In *Textbook of Surgery,* J.D. Hardy (ed.). Philadelphia: Lippincott, 1977. P. 859.

Schindler, R. *Gastroscopy, the Endoscopic Study of Gastric Pathology.* (2nd ed.), New York: Hafner, 1966.

Sugawa, C., et al. Differential topography of acute erosive gastritis due to trauma or sepsis, alcohol or aspirin. *Gastrointest. Endosc.* 19:127, 1973.

Tsuneoka, K., Takemoto, T., and Fukuchi, S. *Fiberscopy of Gastric Diseases.* Baltimore: University Park Press, 1973.

Yamada, T., and Hukuto, M.I. Gastric polyp. *Gastroent. Endosc. (Japan)* 7:448, 1965.

Yoshiaki, I., et al. The endoscopic diagnosis of early gastric cancer. *Gastrointest. Endosc.* 25:96, 1979.

CHAPTER 5

UPPER GASTROINTESTINAL BLEEDING

The flexible esophagogastroduodenoscope finally allowed the clinical management of the patient with upper gastrointestinal bleeding to be put on a rational basis. As long as the physician had to depend on a frequently deceptive clinical history, nonspecific physical findings, and unreliable radiographic reports, the bleeding patient was at an overwhelming disadvantage. Esophagogastroduodenoscopy proved to be a rapid, safe, and reliably informative technique, whether performed in the endoscopy unit or in the emergency room.

PROCEDURES

Most emergency endoscopic examinations are best performed in the endoscopy room or intensive care unit—rather than in the emergency room, where chaos and confusion may be the order of the day or night. Patients who have had recent hematemesis or melena should receive resuscitation immediately to establish reasonably stable vital signs. Prior to endoscopy, the stomach is emptied by gastric lavage with a large-bore Salem sump tube, Ewald tube, or Edlich tube. Although patients may vomit and thus spontaneously evacuate the stomach and esophagus, lavage with ice water is essential to temporarily reduce bleeding. Patients are usually premedicated with intravenous diazepam or meperidine. Cetacaine spray is used to anesthetize the oral pharynx. Marginally stable patients receive only the local analgesic spray as meperidine or diazepam may exacerbate hypotension or hypoventilation. Patients who are in shock, intoxicated, or who have massive arterial bleeding are contraindicated for endoscopic study.

THE ENDOSCOPIC TECHNIQUE

The end-viewing fiberscope is passed through the plastic mouthpiece placed between the patient's teeth or gingivae (see Chapter 3). By having the mouthpiece in place, both the fiberscope and the examiner's finger are spared irreparable damage by a patient who is unable to cooperate fully under these difficult circumstances! The tip of the scope is brought to the base of the tongue, which is pushed forward slightly. The instrument is then advanced into the hypopharynx, keeping it in the midline. The esophagus, esophagogastric junction, body of the stomach, antrum, pylorus, duodenal bulb, and second portion of the duodenum are quickly identified, then systematically examined on withdrawal. Speed is critical in the active bleeder, as the stomach may refill with blood and vision will be obscured. If no bleeding site is found, a U turn maneuver is then performed by bringing the tip of the scope up and sliding it around the greater curvature, to observe the upper greater curvature, fundus, and cardia. Depending on the type of scope and shape of the stomach, the J turn maneuver should also be used by sliding the tip along the lesser curvature to observe the upper lesser curvature, the fundus, and cardia. The patient should be turned onto his right side if blood pools in the fundus, so that the blood will move into the antrum.

When there is special urgency in establishing an early diagnosis in a patient with severe bleeding, endoscopy should be done in the operating room with the patient under general anesthesia, with an endotracheal tube in place. Intraoperative endoscopy will usually reveal the bleeding site because anesthesia decreases splanchnic blood flow, and bleeding has generally decreased sufficiently to allow adequate visualization after gastric lavage. If the abdomen is already open, endoscopy is performed with the proximal jejunum occluded with a noncrushing clamp, to prevent small bowel distention by the insufflated air.

CLINICAL MATERIAL

To enable the student to anticipate the kind of cases he or she may encounter in doing emergency endoscopy for upper gastrointestinal bleeding, the experience at Wayne State University Affiliated Hospitals between November 1971 and December 1978 was analyzed. In this period, 1402 patients with upper gastrointestinal bleeding underwent esophagogastroduodenoscopy (EGD) by members of the Surgical Endoscopic Unit (see Tables 5-1 and 5-2). Complete endoscopic examination was accomplished in 1358 of 1402 patients (97%). Two thousand fifty-six lesions were identified as actual or potential bleeding sites (Table 5-1), caused by erosive gastritis (814), gastric ulcer (261), duodenal ulcer (234), esophageal varices (217), Mallory-Weiss syndrome (161), duodenitis (129), esophagitis (112), gastric tumor (25), gastric varices (21), marginal ulcer (20), and miscellaneous causes (62). The most probable causes of the bleeding are listed in Table 5-2 and are as follows: acute erosive gastritis—503 patients (37%), gastric ulcer—228 (17%), duodenal ulcer—207 patients (15%), Mallory-Weiss syndrome—147 patients (11%), esophageal varices—111 patients (8%), esophagitis—56 patients (4%), duodenitis—25 patients (2%), gastric tumor—24 patients (2%), gastric varices—19 patients (1%), marginal ulcer—18 patients (1%). The endoscopic examination was

Potential Bleeding Site	Number	Active Bleeding Site	%
AGML	814	503	62
Gastric ulcer	261	228	87
Duodenal ulcer	234	207	88
Esophageal varices	217	111	51
Mallory-Weiss syndrome	161	147	91
Duodenitis	129	25	19
Esophagitis	112	56	50
Gastric tumor	25	24	96
Gastric varices	21	19	90
Marginal ulcer	20	18	90
Miscellaneous	62	20	32
Totals	2056	1358	

Table 5-1.   Percentage of Each Identified Lesion That Is the Actual Cause of Bleeding

Source of Bleeding	Number of Patients	%
AGML	503	37
Gastric ulcer	228	17
Duodenal ulcer	207	15
Mallory-Weiss syndrome	147	11
Esophageal varices	111	8
Esophagitis	56	4
Duodenitis	25	2
Gastric tumor	24	2
Gastric varices	19	1
Marginal ulcer	18	1
Miscellaneous	20	2
Totals	1358	100

Table 5-2.   Incidence of Actual Bleeding Sites

not completed in 44 patients because of alcoholic intoxication, inability to negotiate the pylorus, or a hiatal hernia and retained gastric clots.

Erosive Gastritis or Acute Gastric Mucosal Lesions
Alcohol plays a major role in the production of acute gastric mucosal lesions, or AGML, although a significant number of AGML patients also had salicylate exposure. Acute erosive gastritis is characterized by scattered lesions measuring a few millimeters in diameter. They appear as red, black, or white mucosal abrasions, depending on the age of the erosion and whether there is active bleeding. Some of the lesions diag-

nosed endoscopically as erosions might prove to be superficial ulcers extending below the mucosa, if biopsied. The decision to label acute erosive gastritis as the sole source of bleeding can be made only after careful examination of the esophagus, stomach, and duodenum to exclude other possible causes of hemorrhage, as well as by visualizing actual bleeding from the lesion or clots deposited on the erosion.

Gastric Ulcer

An acute gastric ulcer is defined as a shallow crater with a clean base and sharp edges. If examined at the time of bleeding, blood obscures the ulcer or a clot fills the base; careful washing of the suspected area with the Water Pik, which sends a strong, pulsating jet of water down the biopsy channel, is essential. The chronic ulcer has a deep, often shaggy base, and there is swelling of the ulcer edge on which mucosal folds converge. In this study, gastric ulcer proved to be a more common cause of bleeding than duodenal ulcer. Cotton reported that gastric ulcers were the cause of bleeding in 28 percent of the cases as opposed to 24 percent of cases of duodenal ulcer.

Duodenal Ulcer

Duodenal ulcer was the third most frequent cause of bleeding in this series. Twelve percent of the patients with duodenal ulcers were not bleeding from them. Katon and Villar showed a higher incidence of duodenal ulcer bleeding, but this may be due to the difference in patient population and the exclusion of minor gastrointestinal bleeders from their study.

The bleeding duodenal ulcer is frequently difficult to see. The duodenal bulb may be covered with blood, and thus the superficial ulcer cannot be identified. However, when the bleeding can be specifically localized to the bulb, there is little doubt that a duodenal ulcer is responsible for it.

Varices

It is well known that patients with cirrhosis and proven varices are more likely to bleed from another site. In the Wayne State series, however, of the 217 patients with varices, 111 were bleeding from esophageal varices and 19 from gastric varices; i.e., a total of 55 percent of patients. To find actively bleeding varices, early endoscopy is essential (see Plate 42). If immediate endoscopy does not reveal bleeding from esophageal varices, then complete examination of the esophagus, stomach, and duodenum must be done to exclude another site of hemorrhage. Alternating insufflation and suction of air during endoscopy may make the varices more apparent. A discrete blood clot with surrounding ooze of fresh blood on the varix is the usual presentation of variceal rupture, but variceal bleeding can be vigorous at times (Plate 42). The authors do not believe that endoscopy initiates or exacerbates variceal bleeding.

Mallory-Weiss Syndrome

The Mallory-Weiss syndrome describes a mucosal tear on the gastric side of the esophagogastric junction (see Plate 43). Rarely has more than one tear been observed. The laceration characteristically runs parallel to the long axis of the stomach, and may extend proximal to the esophagogastric junction. The bleeding may be arterial or venous, and thus the manifestation may be trivial or catastrophic. Before fiberoptic endoscopy, Mallory-Weiss syndrome was always thought to be a cause of major hemorrhage, only because the diagnosis was usually made in surgery. The incidence of Mallory-Weiss syndrome in the Wayne State series was 11 percent; comparable to the 8 percent reported by Katon and Villar. The Mallory-Weiss syndrome is usually associated with alcohol abuse followed by nausea and vomiting, although some patients have a history of vomiting or severe coughing without prior alcohol ingestion.

Esophagitis

Fifty-six patients (4%) had severe erosive esophagitis as the major source of bleeding. These patients often had associated hiatal hernias, and were elderly or debilitated. Esophagitis typically exhibits diffuse erythematous change of the mucosa as an early stage. White plaques of various configurations surrounded by an erythematous border oozing blood represent a later stage. Diffuse mucosal erosions of the distal esophagus constitute an intermediate stage. Biopsy is not required for this diagnosis, which is obvious endoscopically; tissue is only required to exclude the possibility of cancer.

Duodenitis

Duodenitis caused bleeding in 25 of the 1358 patients (2%) in the Wayne State study. Distal duodenal bulb and proximal descending duodenum were usually observed as the sites for areas of reddened mucosal swelling with scattered superficial erosions. The duodenitis patients had ingested large amounts of alcohol, and very often showed associated pancreatitis. Gelzayd et al. reported that hemorrhagic duodenitis, confirmed by endoscopy and biopsy, accounted for 8 percent of acute upper gastrointestinal bleeders treated by them, an experience not duplicated by other endoscopists.

Neoplasms

Of the twenty gastric tumors found to be the cause of bleeding, twenty were carcinomata, three were leiomyomata, and one was a leiomyosarcoma. In eight of the patients with gastric cancer diagnosed by emergency panendoscopy and biopsy, upper gastrointestinal series performed after endoscopy failed to demonstrate the lesions. Two gastric cancers were less than 2 cm in diameter and relatively superficial.

Marginal Ulcers

Eighteen patients (1%) had bleeding marginal ulcers that were most often found on the jejunal side of the anastomosis. A few cases had deep craters, but usually the ulcers were shallow and contained clots. The upper gastrointestinal series in this group was generally disappointing, giving both false positive and false negative interpretations.

APPROPRIATE TIME FOR ENDOSCOPY

Many studies clearly demonstrate that the diagnostic rate falls significantly as the period between admission and endoscopy lengthens. The authors perform endoscopy in patients with upper gastrointestinal bleeding within 24 hours of admission. No unusual effort is made to do emergency endoscopy, however, except for the massive active gastrointestinal bleeder who is a candidate for emergency surgery. A prudent approach to upper gastrointestinal hemorrhage will yield as good results as the vigorous diagnostic approach, and will reduce the morbidity of the procedure.

Although there is evidence that a careful emergency barium examination, carried out by an experienced radiologist, may produce results rivaling those of endoscopy in identifying chronic deep peptic ulcers, several studies have clearly shown that approximately 30 percent of duodenal ulcers and 40 percent of gastric ulcers will be missed by the standard barium upper gastrointestinal series. The radiologist fails to diagnose almost all acute mucosal lesions. He or she cannot identify a site of bleeding but can only identify a lesion which might be the potential site of bleeding. When an endoscopy failure results because of excessive bleeding, an emergency barium meal will also invariably fail to provide a diagnosis. It is in these patients that arteriography is most likely to show a lesion, and arteriography should be carried out when endoscopy has proved negative or questionable.

ENDOSCOPY IN RELATION TO MANAGEMENT

The value of early diagnosis should not be measured only in terms of reducing mortality from upper gastrointestinal bleeding. Endoscopy facilitates decision-making in medical as well as surgical treatment. Diffuse superficial mucosal lesions are difficult to deal with surgically, while peptic ulcers are amenable to surgery. Endoscopic diagnosis has just about eliminated the need for exploratory gastrotomy or duodenotomy.

Reports assessing the value of early, accurate diagnosis of the bleeding source are conflicting. Surgical postoperative mortality is reduced significantly according to Hoare, but serious disagreement exists regarding the effect of early endoscopic diagnosis on morbidity, duration of hospitalization, and the requirements for blood transfusion. This dispute may never be resolved, however, because of the variety of patient population, variability of associated illnesses, and multitude of causes to be analyzed.

SELECTED READINGS

Allen, H.M., Block, M.A., and Schuman, B.M. Gastroduodenal endoscopy. *Arch. Surg.* 106:450, 1973.

Cotton, P.B., et al. Early endoscopy of oesophagus, stomach, and duodenal bulb in patients with haematemesis and melaena. *Br. Med. J.* 505, 1973.

Donahue, P.E., and Nyhus, L.M. Massive Upper Gastrointestinal Hemorrhage. In L.M. Nyhus and C. Wastell (eds.), *Surgery of the Stomach and Duodenum.* Boston: Little, Brown, 1977. P. 405.

Eastwood, G.L. Does early endoscopy benefit the patient with active upper gastrointestinal bleeding? *Gastroenterology* 72:737, 1977.

Forrest, J.A.H., and Finlayson, N.D.C. Endoscopy in gastrointestinal bleeding. *Lancet* 394, 1974.

Gelzayd, E.A., and Gelfand, D.W. Hemorrhagic duodenitis: A significant cause of gastrointestinal bleeding. *Gastrointest. Endosc.* 20:59, 1973.

Hoare, A.M. Comparative study between endoscopy and radiology in acute upper gastrointestinal hemorrhage. *Br. Med. J.* 27, 1975.

Katon, R.M., and Smith, F.W. Panendoscopy in the early diagnosis of acute upper gastrointestinal bleeding. *Gastroenterology* 65:728, 1973.

Katz, D. Endoscopy in upper gastrointestinal bleeding: Then and now. *Gastrointest. Endosc.* 21:109, 1975.

Knauer, C.M. Mallory-Weiss syndrome. Characterization of 75 Mallory-Weiss lacerations in 528 patients with upper gastrointestinal hemorrhage. *Gastroenterology* 71:5, 1976.

Lucas, C.E., and Sugawa, C. Diagnostic endoscopy during laparotomy for acute hemorrhage from the upper part of the gastrointestinal tract. *Surg. Gynecol. Obstet.* 135:285, 1972.

McGinn, F.P., Guyer, P.B., and Wilkin, B.J. A prospective comparative trial between early endoscopy and radiology in acute upper gastrointestinal hemorrhage. *Gut* 16:707, 1975.

Sugawa, C., et al. Early endoscopy: A guide to therapy for acute upper gastrointestinal hemorrhage. *Arch. Surg.* 107:133, 1973.

Villar, H.V., et al. Emergency diagnosis of upper gastrointestinal bleeding by fiberoptic endoscopy. *Ann. Surg.* 185:367, 1977.

Waldram, R., et al. Emergency endoscopy after gastrointestinal hemorrhage in 50 patients with portal hypertension. *Br. Med. J.* 4:94, 1974.

ENDOSCOPIC RETROGRADE CHOLANGIO-PANCREATOGRAPHY

INSTRUMENTS

Endoscopic cannulation of the ampulla of Vater was first described by McCune in 1968. Since the development of a side-viewing duodenoscope in Japan by the Machida Manufacturing Company and the Olympus Optical Company in 1969, the technique of cannulation has been widely employed by endoscopists throughout the world.

Since 1972 the authors have been using the Olympus duodenoscope, which has become (in the United States) the standard instrument for cannulation. The Olympus fiberduodenoscope (JF-B1, JF-B2, and JF-B3) (see Fig. 6-1) is equipped with a side-viewing optical system, and has a working length of 125 cm and a diameter of 10 mm. The short movable tip (46 mm long) deflects 120 degrees up and down, and 90 degrees right and left. The forceps elevator enables the operator to adjust the elevation angle of the cannula, cytology brush, or biopsy forceps to a maximum of 80 degrees. The fingertip valves control air, water, and suction. The side-viewing lens allows a field of vision of 65 degrees, with the fixed focus giving a range of observation from 5 to 60 mm.

A Teflon cannula (JF-B3, 1.7 mm in diameter) is marked with three 3-mm bands at the tip. A 5 French biopsy forceps is available and cytology can be done with a nylon brush pushed through the biopsy channel. Olympus CLE and CLS light sources are sufficient for routine use, but high-intensity light provided by model CLX is necessary to make movies and videotapes (see Fig. 6-2).

PREPARATION OF THE PATIENT

Most patients have already been hospitalized before the procedure, but endoscopic retrograde cholangiopancreatography (ERCP) may be performed on an outpatient basis for the anicteric patients. Where no obstruction or stricture of the biliary tract or pancreatic duct is evident after successful cannulation, the patient need not be hospitalized. If ERCP is scheduled in the morning, the patient should receive nothing by mouth after the preceding midnight. But if the procedure is to be done in the afternoon, a clear liquid breakfast is permitted at seven.

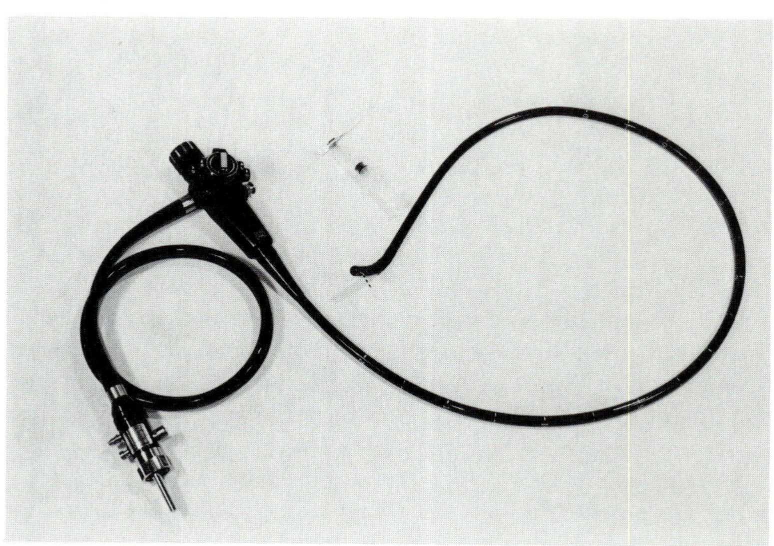

Figure 6-1. The Olympus JF-B3 duodenoscope. The cannula for retrograde injection protrudes from the biopsy channel.

Medication

Intramuscular premedication consisting of atropine (0.4–0.6 mg) and meperidine (50–75 mg) is given about 30 minutes prior to examination. After the scout film is taken, Cetacaine Spray is applied to the oral pharynx, and an antiforming agent is given orally, or with irrigation water through the endoscope. Diazepam (2.5–10.0 mg) is given slowly through an already established intravenous infusion line in the right arm. Intravenous diazepam (2.5–10.0 mg) or meperidine (25–50 mg) is given additionally in patients who are still restless. A dose of 0.4 mg atropine or an anticholinergic agent such as tridihexethyl chloride (Pathilon) may be given a few minutes before the procedure to control peristalsis and relax smooth muscle. Glucagon (0.25–0.5 mg) is given intravenously as the papilla comes into view to relax the Vaterian muscle. Additional doses of these medications are given as often as needed in small increments during the procedure, which may last up to an hour.

Contrast Media

The authors use Renografin (a 60% and 30% solution of meglumine diatrizoate and sodium diatrizoate respectively), but other contrast agents may be used such as Hypaque sodium 50%, Conray (60%), and Vascoray. If the biliary tree is to be examined for calculi, contrast (diluted with equal amounts of saline) should be available so as to allow visualization of small calculi. The authors routinely

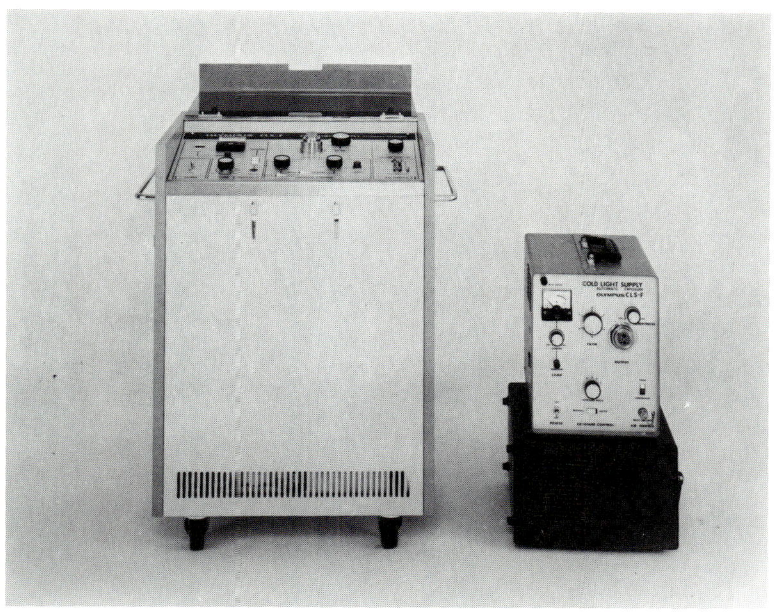

Figure 6-2. CLX-F and CLS-F light sources from Olympus Corporation.

add 80 mg of gentamicin to the syringe containing 50 cc of Renografin.

INDICATIONS

Many problems of diagnosis and management of pancreatic and biliary disease can be resolved by radiographic studies obtained from cannulation of the ampulla of Vater. In addition, a variety of procedures may be performed, such as the collection of pancreatic fluid for cytology and biochemical studies, the measurement of sphincteric pressure, and papillotomy.

Indications for ERCP can be divided into the following categories: (1) jaundice of undetermined etiology, (2) suspected biliary tract disease without jaundice, (3) suspected or known pancreatic disease.

Indications for ERCP
  I. Jaundice of undetermined etiology
     A. Demonstration of extrahepatic biliary obstruction
        1. Stones
        2. Primary and secondary neoplasm
        3. Stricture
        4. Sclerosing cholangitis
        5. Papillary stenosis

     B. Demonstration of normal extrahepatic biliary tract in suspected intrahepatic cholestasis
II. Suspected biliary tract disease without jaundice
     A. Stones in bile ducts or gallbladder
     B. Pancreatitis
     C. Postcholecystectomy syndrome
        1. Dilatation
        2. Stricture
        3. Retained stone
III. Suspected or known pancreatic disease
     A. Pancreatitis
        1. Acute recurrent
        2. Chronic
        3. Pseudocyst
     B. Neoplasm
        1. Benign
        2. Malignant
     C. Evaluation of the duct before and after pancreatic surgery
     D. Developmental anomaly
        1. Pancreas divisum
        2. Annular pancreas

Jaundice of Undetermined Etiology

A case with jaundice becomes a difficult diagnostic problem when the usual tests fail to distinguish between intra- and extrahepatic obstruction. If the patient with intrahepatic obstruction is mistakenly operated on, surgery may precipitate liver failure and bring about a protracted course, or lethal outcome. It is obviously desirable to operate on the patient with extrahepatic obstruction to perform a definitive therapeutic procedure before the obstruction itself leads to liver failure. ERCP is a diagnostic modality that allows establishment of the etiology of jaundice in the early stages of illness. Moreover, the surgeon can proceed with preoperative knowledge of the anatomy of the biliary system, as well as of the exact location of the obstructing lesion.

Suspected Biliary Tract Disease Without Jaundice

There are a number of patients with symptoms suggestive of biliary tract disease in whom routine investigative methods have yielded negative or equivocal results. ERCP is an invaluable technique to confirm or disprove the biliary tract pathology. Patients who complain of persistent epigastric or right upper quadrant pain after cholecystectomy may have common bile duct (CBD) stones, stricture, or pancreatitis. A normal pancreatogram or cholangiogram is obviously very useful in the management of this group of patients, and avoids unnecessary operations.

Suspected or Known Pancreatic Disease
ERCP is important in the diagnosis of pancreatic disease because it often provides precise anatomic information in cases of chronic and relapsing pancreatitis, pseudocyst, pancreatic cancer, and developmental anomaly such as pancreas divisum. If the clinical situation warrants corrective surgery, a pancreatogram is essential in preoperative planning for surgical therapy of chronic pancreatitis.

CONTRAINDICATIONS AND COMPLICATIONS
Contraindications and complications of ERCP are similar to those of any upper gastrointestinal endoscopic procedure as discussed in other chapters. The complications that relate specifically to ERCP follow successful cannulation and the filling of ducts with contrast material.

The most frequent complications of ERCP are benign asymptomatic hyperamylasemia and hyperamylasuria, which persist 24 to 48 hours in the absence of pain. Pancreatitis caused by excessive injection pressure and characterized by epigastric pain lasting more than two hours is associated with hyperamylasemia and hyperamylasuria, low grade fever, and leucocytosis. This type of pancreatitis responds rapidly to conservative management and is not associated with significant morbidity or mortality. Pancreatic sepsis and pseudocyst abscess are serious complications with appreciable mortality. Septic complications occur when contrast material passes beyond an obstruction or fills a nondraining cystic cavity. ERCP should not be performed unless the patient's condition is good enough to permit surgical correction of any obstruction, lesion, or pseudocyst that might be found. Cholangitis is a relatively infrequent but severe complication that occurs only when there is biliary tract obstruction due to either a tumor or calculi. ERCP should be done in the event of the bile duct obstruction only when the patient is a candidate for early surgical relief of the obstruction. The success rate of cannulation increases and the complication rate decreases with the experience of the examiner.

THE TECHNIQUE OF ERCP
There are three obstacles to successful completion of ERCP. The first is intubation of the pylorus with the side-viewing duodenoscope. The second is the identification of the papilla, and the third is cannulation of

the papilla to achieve opacification of the biliary tract and pancreatic duct.

To get over these hurdles, the endoscopist must insure that the patient is well motivated and relaxed. Motivation is achieved by a reasonably complete discussion of the technique, possible discomfort involved, and length of the procedure. This discussion also includes an appraisal of the risk of complications in that particular patient, but of course the risk varies depending on whether the patient is being examined for obstructive jaundice, chronic pancreatitis, or unexplained pain. Even the best-motivated patient requires adequate medication to be relaxed during the procedure which, in a difficult case, may take up to an hour to complete. Appropriate premedication as well as intermittent intravenous medication during the procedure must be given, although there are a few patients who do remarkably well with little or no analgesia or sedation.

The lateral-viewing duodenoscope, being of smaller diameter than the standard forward-viewing duodenoscope, is usually passed without difficulty through the mouthpiece to the back of the tongue. Then with the lateral flexion locked, a small amount of vertical flexion will pass the tip of the instrument to the cricopharyngeus, which generally will yield with a swallow for passage into the esophagus and stomach. Following insufflation of air, the angulus is readily identified and the pylorus brought into view. At this point it is wise to be sure that there is no loop of the scope in the stomach by pulling back on the instrument. When the pylorus is in view, the duodenoscope is then advanced with the right hand, and the tip is raised slightly as the pylorus moves into the six o'clock position. With rotation of the shaft of the instrument in a clockwise manner, the pylorus will be passed and the instrument will generally move out of the bulb into the descending duodenum. Again, the scope should be pulled back to remove any loop that has formed within the stomach, so that passage into the descending duodenum is performed with as straight a duodenoscope as possible.

Once the transverse folds of the descending duodenum are identified, the patient is then moved from the left lateral decubitus position to the prone position. At this point an intravenous anticholinergic agent is given to reduce peristalsis in the duodenum but sometimes, if the pylorus has been unusually spastic, it may have to be given earlier to relax the pylorus.

The search for the papilla begins on withdrawal from the distal descending duodenum. The papilla of Vater will usually be found at the 10-to-12 o'clock position in the midportion of the descending duodenum, although it is more commonly closer to the proximal third of the distal descending duodenum than the distal third. One should look for a vertical fold that traverses the transverse folds and if found, trace it to its proximal (usually bulbous) end. There the papilla is most often located, although the papilla may be anywhere on that fold (see Fig. 6-3). Unfortunately, the vertical fold is not invariably present, and the papilla can only be found by identification of somewhat subtle mucosal changes. The surface of the papilla often looks as if it has been salted, and a red point may be evident in a central position. The diameter of the papilla is quite variable. The papilla may be flat or may actually bulge into the lumen like a nipple. If glucagon is given at this time, a flat papilla will not infrequently change its contour and become somewhat bulbous. If the papilla is small and has neither mucoid spotting nor a fold like a monk's hood over its superior border, then you are probably dealing with the minor papilla, and the major papilla should be found 1 to 3 cm below.

In order to cannulate the papilla, it must be viewed directly on a frontal view. To attempt to cannulate from a tangential point or at too great a distance is simply wasting time. Various maneuvers will permit this en face approach to the papilla. The most obvious correction is to change the tip direction. If this does not succeed, advancing or withdrawing the tip may bring the papilla into better view (see Fig. 6-4A,B). Putting torsion on the shaft of the instrument by rotation, either clockwise or counterclockwise, may also be worthwhile. Finally, changing the position of the patient to the left lateral decubitus position may be required, as may be, in some circumstances, actually supporting the patient so that he or she is turned slightly onto his or her back. Once the papilla is brought into appropriate alignment, it must be kept in view at all times as the catheter is passed down the biopsy channel. To lose the papilla at this point may mean the loss of much time in reestablishing the appropriate position.

When the tip of the catheter is in sight, it is directed to the point of the papilla where an orifice has been identified. While the catheter is

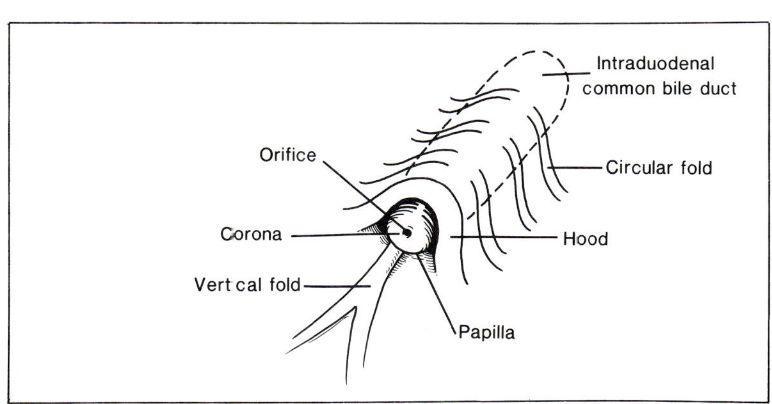

Figure 6-3. Normal anatomy of the ampulla of Vater.

Figure 6-4. *Roentgenograms showing position of the duodenoscope in the approach to the papilla. A. Large loop along the greater curvature of the stomach is reduced as shown in B.*

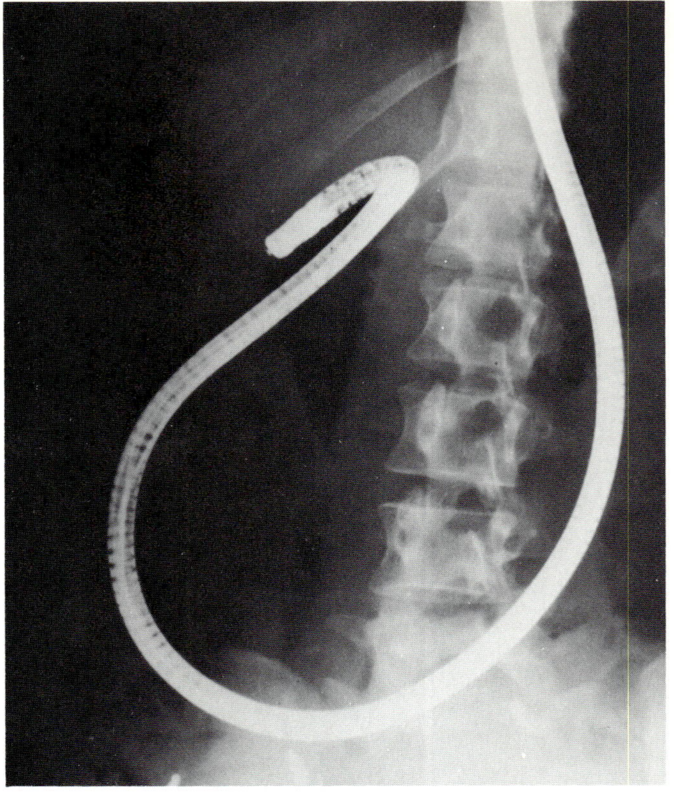

A

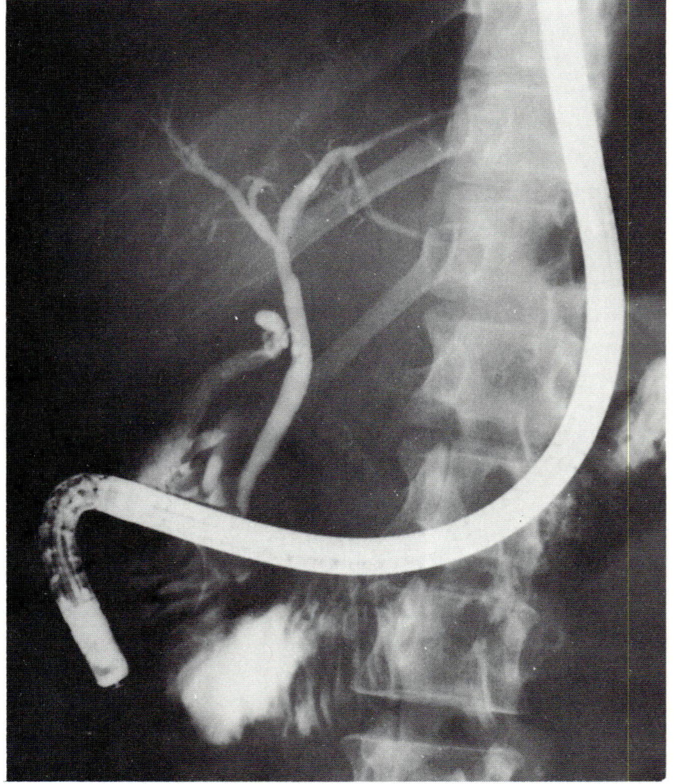

B

being passed down the biopsy channel, the examiner should have studied carefully the surface of the papilla to identify the orifice and to exclude the possibility of a second orifice. The ductal orifice is generally central, slightly depressed, and somewhat reddened. If bile is seen to trickle from that area, there is no question of the location. If no orifice can be identified, then it is best to start centrally and work around the surface of the papilla in a methodical fashion, with the hope of finally entering the orifice.

The cannula should not be jammed into the orifice, but gently insinuated. Once the first 2-mm mark is within the indentation of the orifice, then the instrument tip should be reoriented so that the cannula is not going in at an angle. To determine whether the cannula is impacted into the orifice, 3 or 4 ml of contrast is injected under fluoroscopic control until either leakage of contrast fluid into the duodenum is evident or ductal opacification occurs. If the pancreatic duct is visualized, then further injection is made to obtain opacification of the tail of the pancreatic duct. Spot films then must be taken of the pancreatic duct at the time of the filling since the pancreatic duct, if not grossly abnormal, will empty promptly and a postinjection film will not show the whole duct.

One should always attempt to get opacification of both duct systems and, since the pancreatic duct fills in a higher percentage of cases than does the biliary duct, one is usually in the position of redirecting the cannula after pancreatography to inject the common bile duct. The first maneuver under these circumstances is to withdraw the cannula as far as possible without its falling out of the orifice. The physician should then reinject on the expectation that he or she is dealing with a common channel, and that both ducts can be filled at the same time if the injection is made at the very distal end of the ampulla. If this fails, one must engage the tip of the cannula in the orifice and advance the cannula so that it bends downward, causing the tip to angle upward. This maneuver attempts to take advantage of the fact that the common bile duct comes into the ampulla from an angle of approximately 45 degrees in relation to the pancreatic duct. If this also fails, then one must assume that both ducts exit at the orifice and are separated by a septum that protects the bile duct. The roofing technique as described by Vennes involves withdrawing the cannula to the orifice and then, with a forceful upward push, attempting to override the septum and pass into the common bile duct. Should all these maneuvers fail, then one should look again for a second orifice. The common bile duct orifice usually resides above and to the left of the pancreatic orifice. If cannulation has failed after one hour of procedural time, it is best to stop the procedure and bring the patient back for a second try at a later date when, surprisingly, cannulation may proceed with considerable rapidity for unknown reasons.

In patients who have had subtotal gastrectomy, the technique obviously must be different. Where there is a gastroduodenoscopy, the papilla is often found quite close to the stoma. Where there is a gastrojejunostomy, the papilla may be more easily identified with a forward-viewing instrument (see Fig. 6-5); indeed, the small caliber pediatric instruments have been found to be useful under these circumstances.

Where a sphincteroplasty has been done or a choledochoduodenostomy has been performed, cannulation is generally quite easy, but it should be remembered that the patient must be supine in the head-down position to retain contrast in the intrahepatic ducts.

The ERCP procedure is a very satisfying examination when it provides exact, indisputable radiographic evidence for a correct diagnosis. The procedure can also be very frustrating due to factors beyond the endoscopist's control. Obviously where pyloric stenosis exists, intubation of the duodenum will fail in many instances. The presence of duodenal diverticula makes cannulation difficult or impossible when the papilla is out of sight in the diverticulum. Frequently cannulation is

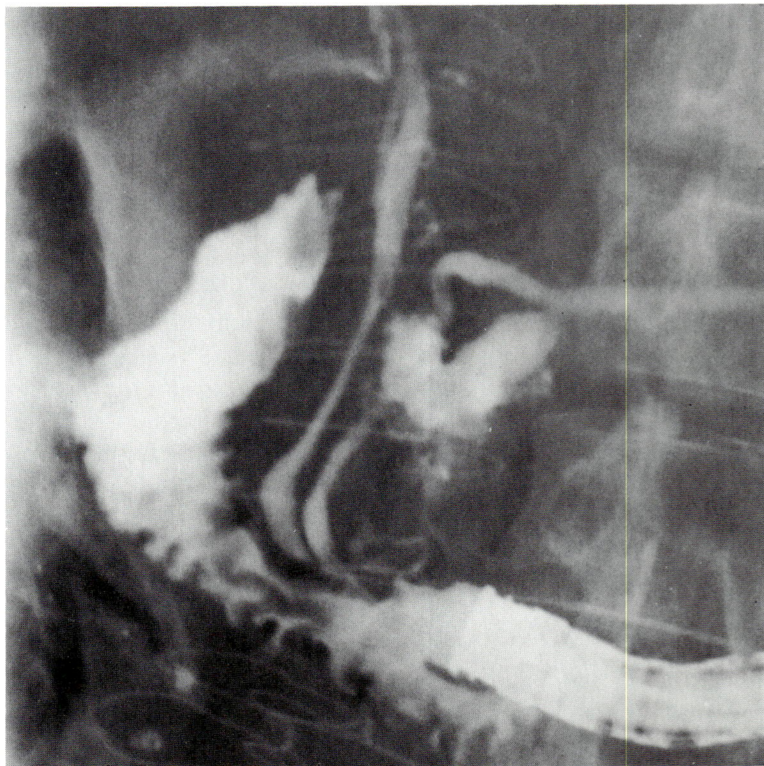

Figure 6-5.   Forward-viewing gastroduodenoscope (GIF-D) used for cannulation of the papilla via the afferent loop of a Billroth II anastomosis. Both common bile duct and pancreatic duct are opacified, and a pseudocyst fills from the pancreatic duct. (From C. Sugawa and A. J. Walt, Endoscopic retrograde pancreatography in the surgery of pancreatic pseudocysts. Surgery *86: 643, 1979. Reprinted courtesy of the C.V. Mosby Company.)*

unsuccessful because of the nature of the pathology, and in patients with chronic pancreatitis or distal ampullary disease it will not be possible to inject contrast material, although usually there are endoscopic findings to explain these failures. In the majority of cases, however, an experienced endoscopist can accomplish successful cannulation of a duct within the first 20 minutes of the examination.

Results

The experience between 1972 and 1977 at Henry Ford Hospital and Wayne State University Hospitals (in Michigan) involved 1044 patients who underwent ERCP. The age range was from 12 to 90 years. The female to male ratio was 1.0 to 1.3. Diagnosis was made by ERCP in 82.2 percent of the patients.

JAUNDICE.   Of the 371 patients tabulated here, 119 had a normal common bile duct or pancreatic duct, or both.

Carcinoma of pancreas	80
Nonsurgical jaundice	119
Choledocholithiasis	43
Narrowing of common bile duct	38
Periampullary cancer	10
Carcinoma of bile ducts	12
Sclerosing cholangitis	3
Choledochal cyst	3
Narrowing of choledochoduodenostomy	1
Unsuccessful	62
Total number of patients	371

The normal biliary tract is characterized by homogeneous filling of the extrahepatic bile duct, gallbladder, and intrahepatic duct (see Fig. 6-6). The cystic duct may join the common bile duct (CBD) at any level above the sphincter of Oddi. Intrahepatic jaundice is established by excluding extrahepatic obstruction. Five patients had incidental gallbladder stones with normal-caliber common bile and hepatic duct consistent with intrahepatic jaundice (see Fig. 6-7).

Carcinoma of the head of the pancreas was found in 80 patients. In eight patients there was invasion of the pancreatic tumor in the descending duodenum. The diagnosis of pancreatic cancer can be made either by cholangiography, by pancreatography, or both.

Stones in the CBD have been cited as the most frequent cause of extrahepatic biliary obstruction, and this was found in 43 of our cases (see Fig. 6-8). Some stones impacted at the sphincter of Oddi can float up into the bile duct when cannulation is done, and bile may flow more freely (see Fig. 6-9A,B). Sludge (sand) may be found by careful fluoroscopy and multiple spot films during various stages of filling of

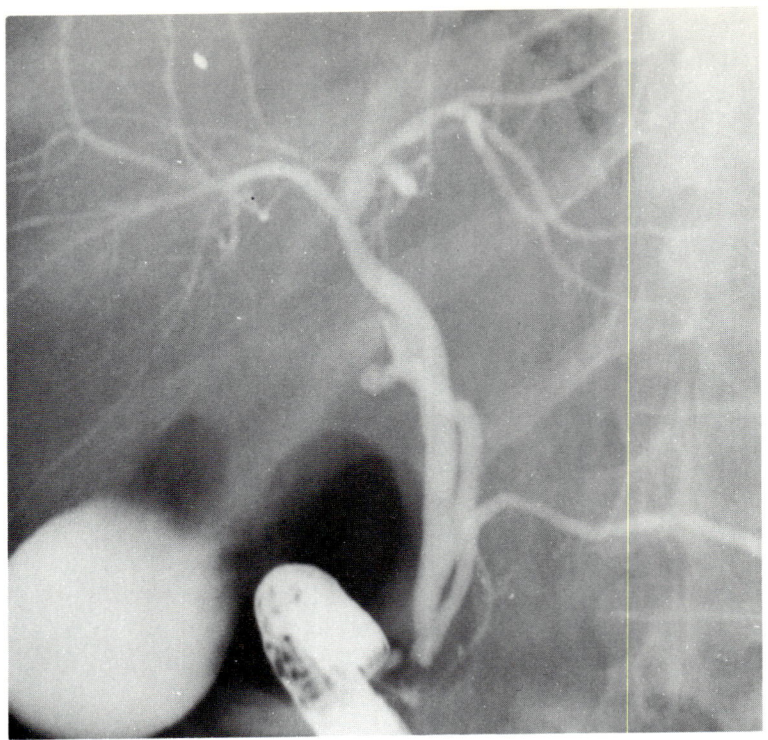

Figure 6-6. Normal biliary tract. The cystic duct joins the common duct distally. The gallbladder is in the right lower corner of the picture. The pancreatic duct crosses the vertebral spine.

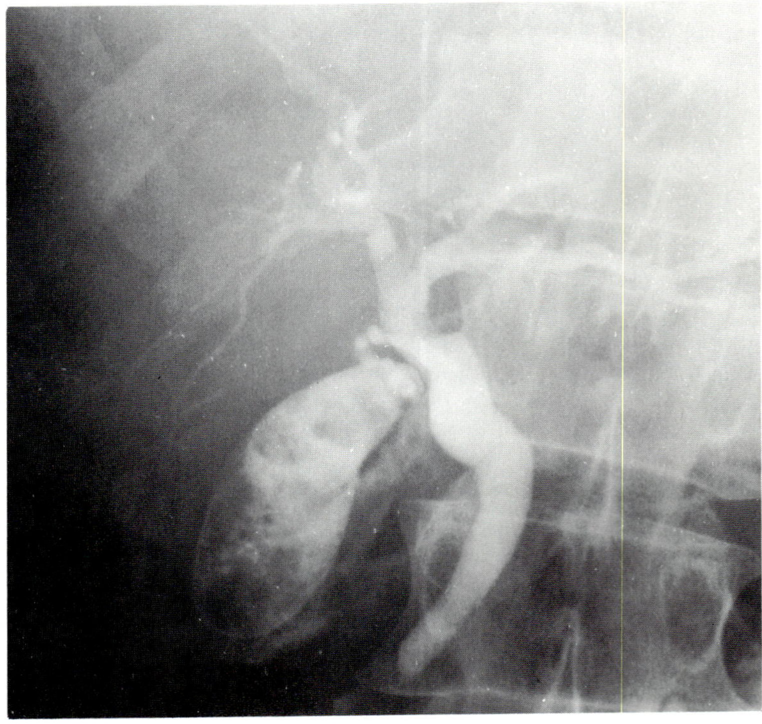

Figure 6-7. These are multiple large stones in the gallbladder. There is no obstruction to bile flow. The cystic duct is narrow.

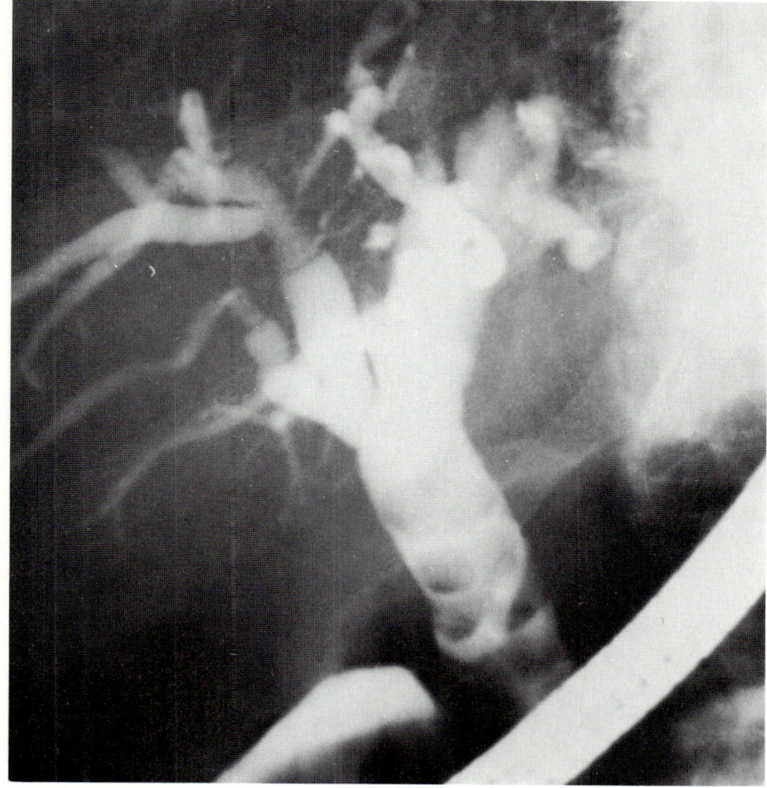

Figure 6-8.   Several stones are present in the dilated common bile duct.

the biliary tree with contrast; this finding may account for jaundice although no definite calculi are present.

Narrowing of the common bile duct may be caused by papillary stenosis and benign stricture after biliary surgery and pancreatitis. Twenty-five patients had a narrowing at the ampulla of Vater; seven patients had a stricture at the distal common bile duct due to pancreatitis (see Fig. 6-10). Six patients were noted to have a stricture at the level of a cystic duct remnant after cholecystectomy (see Fig. 6-11).

Carcinoma of the biliary tract, although not very common, should be in the differential diagnosis of jaundice. Twelve patients were shown to have carcinoma of the biliary tract both primary and secondary (see Fig. 6-12).

Radiologic features encountered with ERCP in biliary tract cancer include

1. Stenosis of the bile duct system with dilatation of the upper duct system and its branches, and a normal appearance of the duct below the site of obstruction

Figure 6-9.   A. Retained stone after cholecystectomy. B. The retained stone has been pushed up into the left hepatic duct by the injection of contrast material.

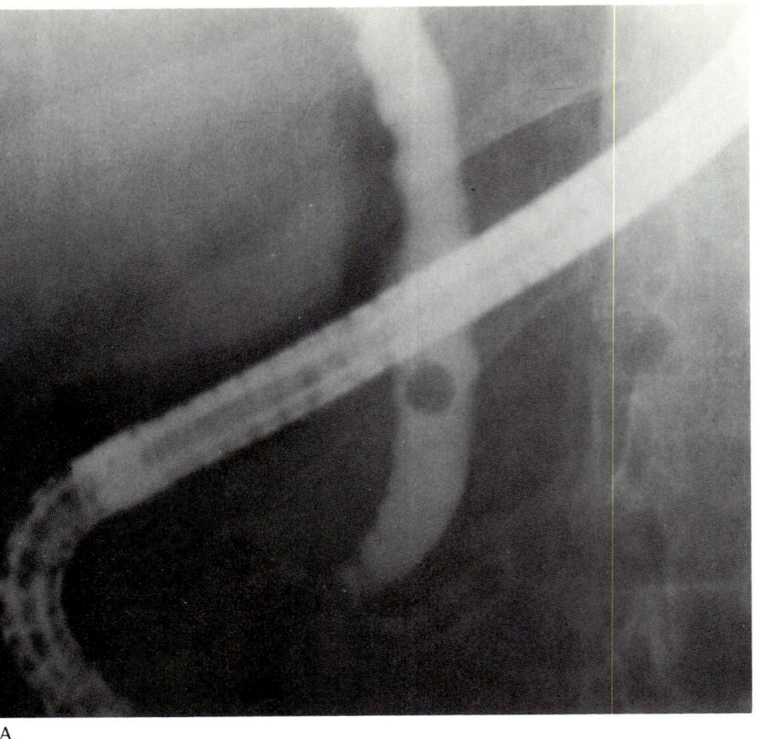

A

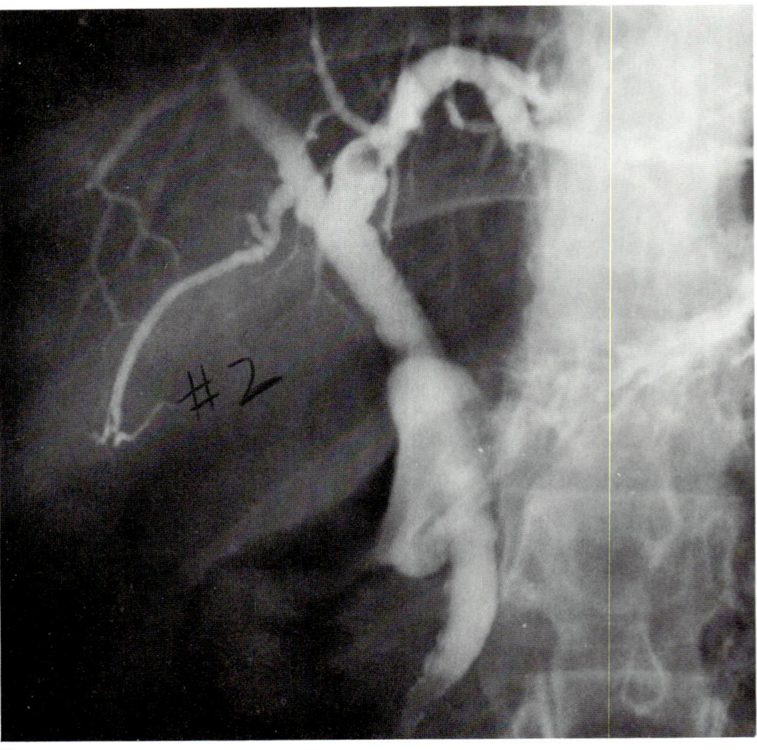

B

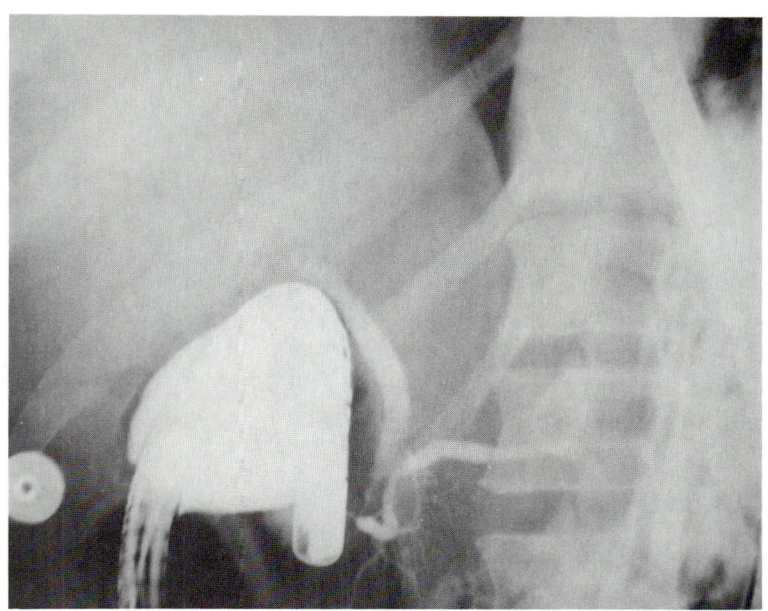

Figure 6-10.   Narrowing of the distal common bile duct by chronic pancreatitis. The pancreatic duct is narrow in the head where it is adjacent to the common bile duct.

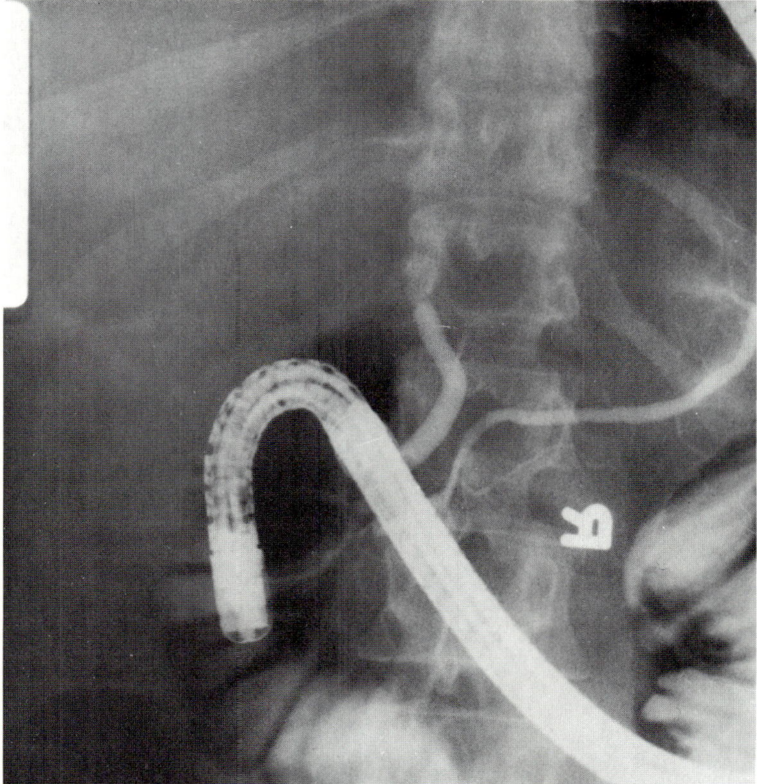

Figure 6-11.   A stricture is present at the level of the cystic duct junction.

Figure 6-12. The irregular narrowing of the midcommon bile duct is consistent with primary cancer.

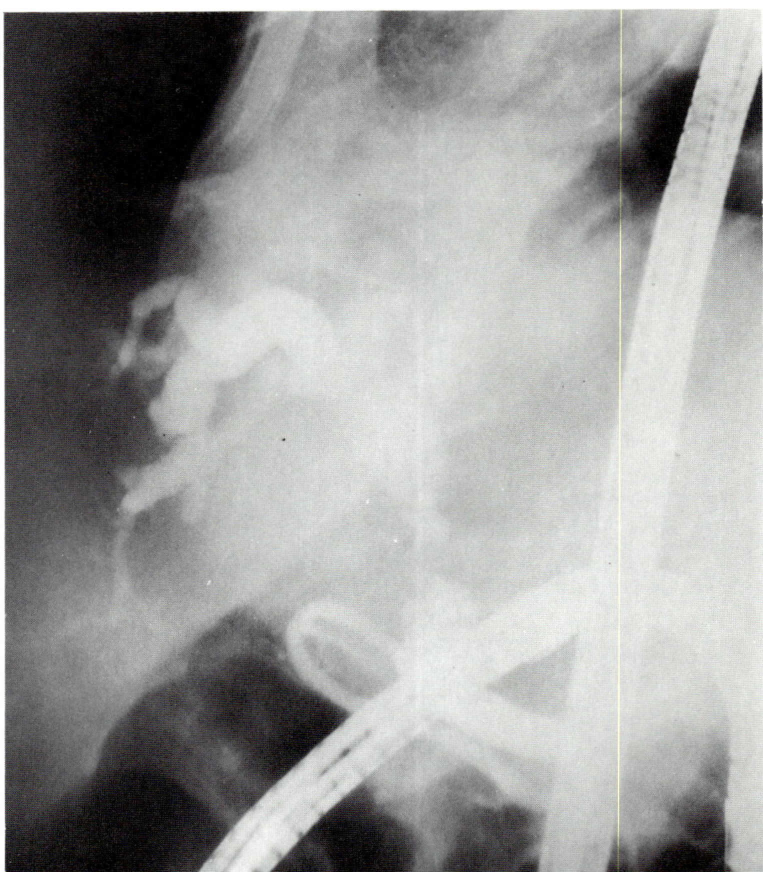

2. Abrupt blockage of the common bile duct with irregular ragged contour
3. Complete stenosis of one of the hepatic ducts without filling of its branches

There were ten patients with periampullary cancer. The papilla of Vater is usually enlarged and may have a lobulated surface with an occasional ulceration. Multiple biopsies are very important in order to establish an accurate diagnosis. The ductogram often shows only the narrowing at the ampulla of Vater (see Fig. 6–13), but in advanced stages the extension of the tumor can be identified on the x-ray film.

Three patients had sclerosing cholangitis. All three patients showed irregular and shaggy contour of the extrahepatic duct with focal strictures (see Fig. 6–14). The intrahepatic ducts revealed marked pruning and stenosis. Primary sclerosing cholangitis develops spontaneously as

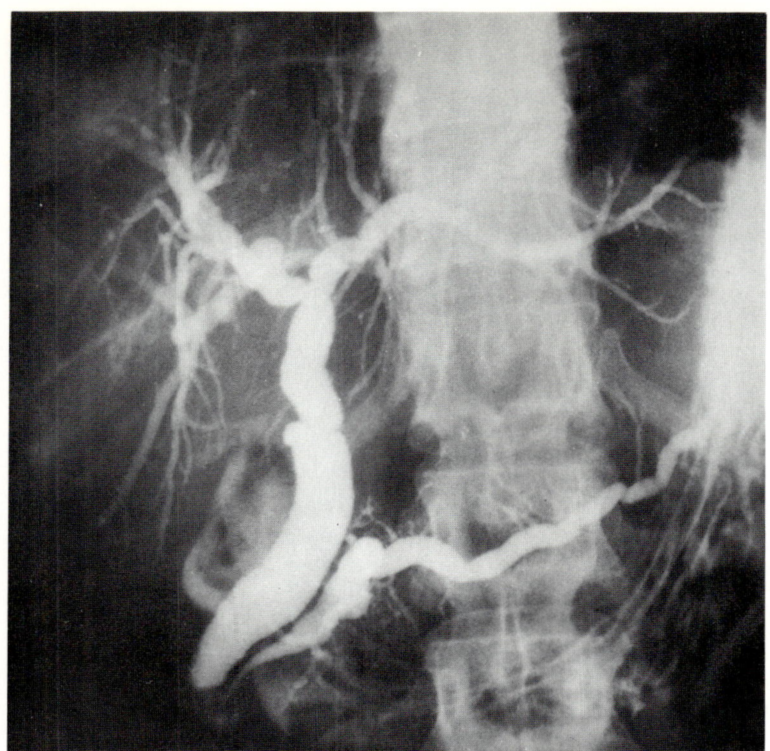

Figure 6-13.   Minimal dilation of both the common bile duct and pancreatic duct. The obstruction was proven by biopsy to be due to a small carcinoma of the ampulla.

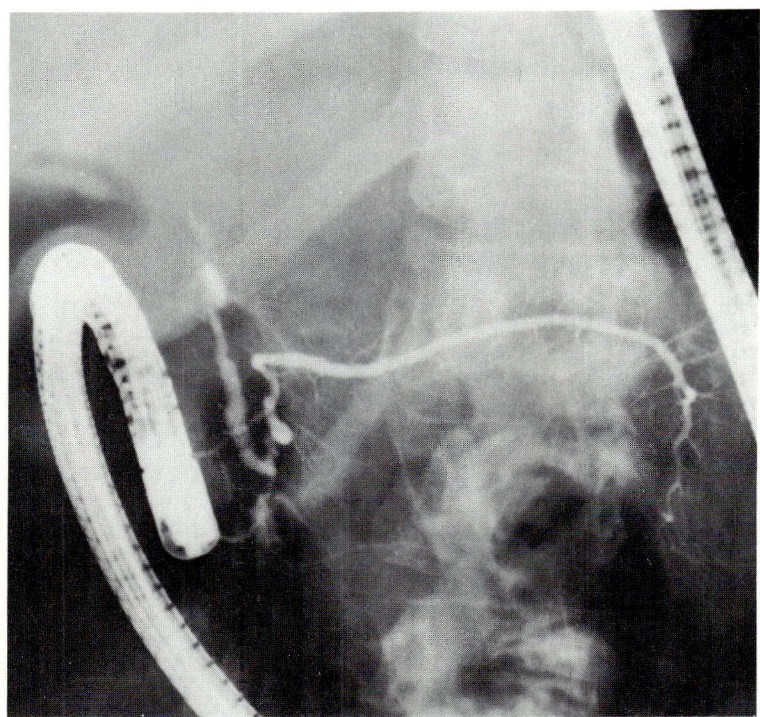

Figure 6-14.   The irregular contour of the common bile duct is characteristic of cholangitis. The pancreatic duct is normal.

in these cases, or it can be associated with ulcerative or granulomatous colitis.

Choledochal cysts were found in three patients. All the cysts were located in the distal common bile duct.

Suspected Biliary Tract Disease Without Jaundice
One hundred twenty-one patients had complained of persistent unexplained epigastric or right upper quadrant pain.

Normal	44
Narrowing of CBD	16
Choledocholithiasis	12
Cholelithiasis	8
Pancreatitis	18
Bile leakage	1
Unsuccessful	21
Total number of patients	121

Most of these patients had had a cholecystectomy and, in all cases tested, intravenous cholangiograms were normal or inconclusive. There was an abnormality by ERCP in 55 cases including CBD stones, gallbladder stones, cystic duct remnant, and stricture (see Fig. 6-15). ERCP showed a stricture and leakage of the bile duct at the cystic duct stump in one patient who continued to leak a large amount of the bile from the drain site for a month after cholecystectomy (see Fig. 6-16).

Suspected Pancreatic Disease
The diagnosis established by ERCP is summarized below.

Pancreatitis	169
Pseudocyst	60
Normal	168
Carcinoma	28
Pancreas divisum	8
Cholelithiasis	13
Miscellaneous	4
Ampullary cancer	1
Unsuccessful	101
Total number of patients	552

Of 552 patients with suspected pancreatic disease, 168 had a normal pancreatic duct, common bile duct, or both. The normal pancreatogram shows considerable variation, and it is difficult to establish rigid criteria for the normal pancreatic duct system. The ductal configura-

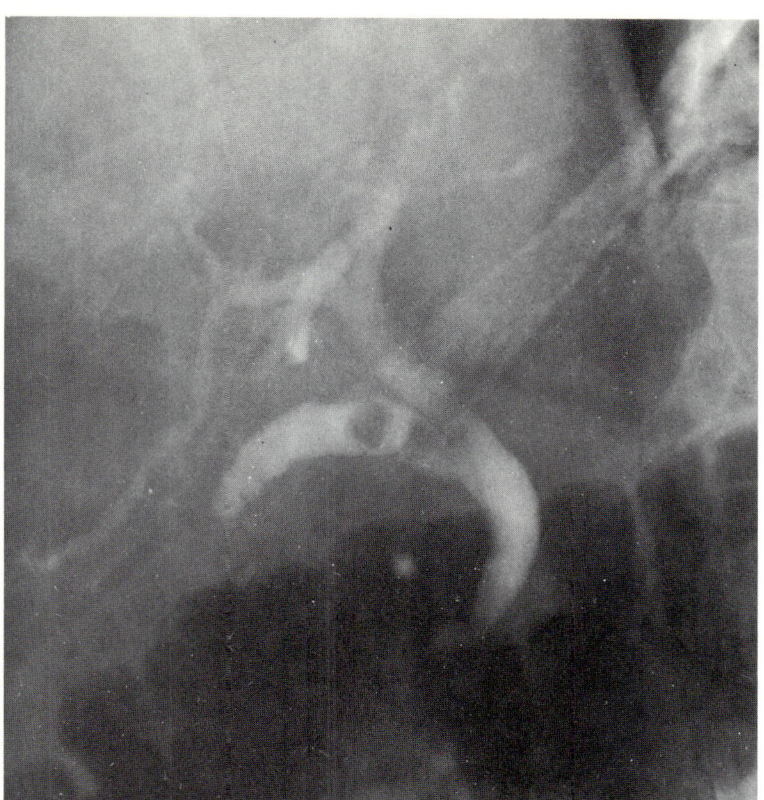

Figure 6-15. Two stones are present in a long cystic duct remnant.

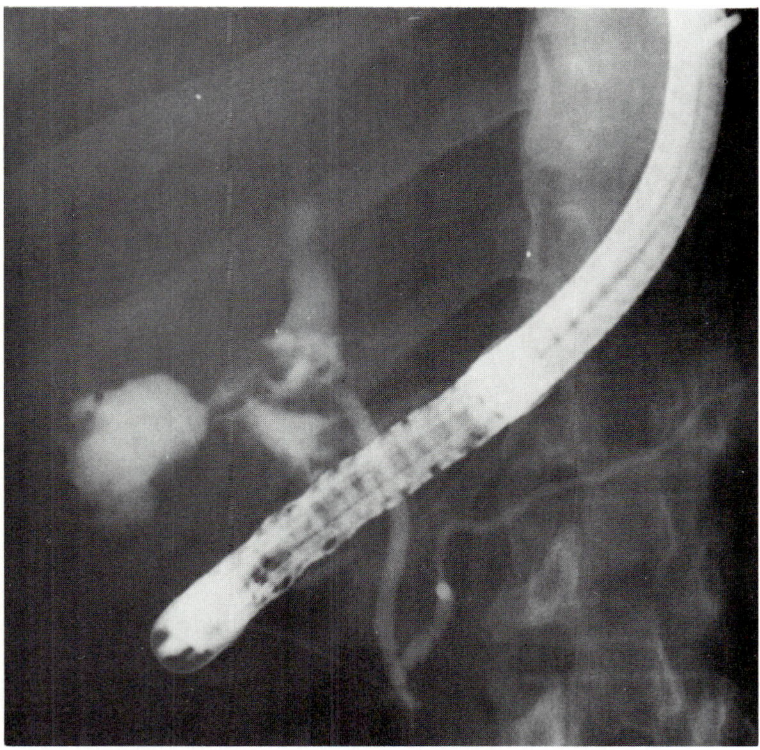

Figure 6-16. Contrast material extravasates from a site above a stricture at the level of the cystic duct junction. The proximal common hepatic duct is dilated.

tion in the head may be quite variable, depending on the level and direction at which dorsal and ventral branches anastomose to form the adult pancreatic duct. Depending on the amount of injected contrast material, the main pancreatic duct, lateral branches, and acini will be filled out and depicted. Usually the normal pancreatic duct tapers gently from the head to the tail, diminishing in diameter from 3 mm to 1 mm respectively. Thin lateral branches project at irregular intervals from the duct (see Fig. 6-17).

CHRONIC PANCREATITIS.   Chronic pancreatitis was found in 169 patients. Chronic pancreatitis may elude diagnosis by means of retrograde pancreatography because the severity or duration of disease may not be reflected by ductal changes. Anacker et al. have categorized pancreatitis in three stages ranging from minimal ductal alteration to marked changes of the ductal system.

Stage 1: Minimal Abnormality. There is irregularity in width at the side branches of the main pancreatic duct resulting from fibrosis of the pancreatic parenchyma. Areas of mild proximal dilatation or cystic change may be observed; this may be diffuse or localized. The main duct of the pancreas shows slight marginal irregularities (see Fig. 6-18).

Stage 2: Moderate Abnormality. As the disease progresses, significant areas of narrowing and dilatation occur in the main duct as well as in the branches (see Fig. 6-19).

Stage 3: Advanced Abnormality. Severe changes of the entire ductal system are found. Gross areas of stricture, dilatation, and tortuosity

Figure 6-17.   A normal pancreatic duct.

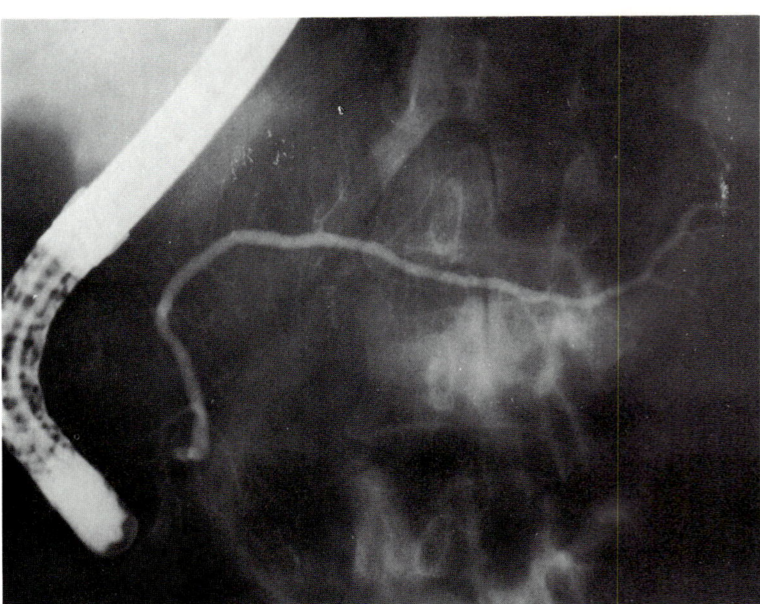

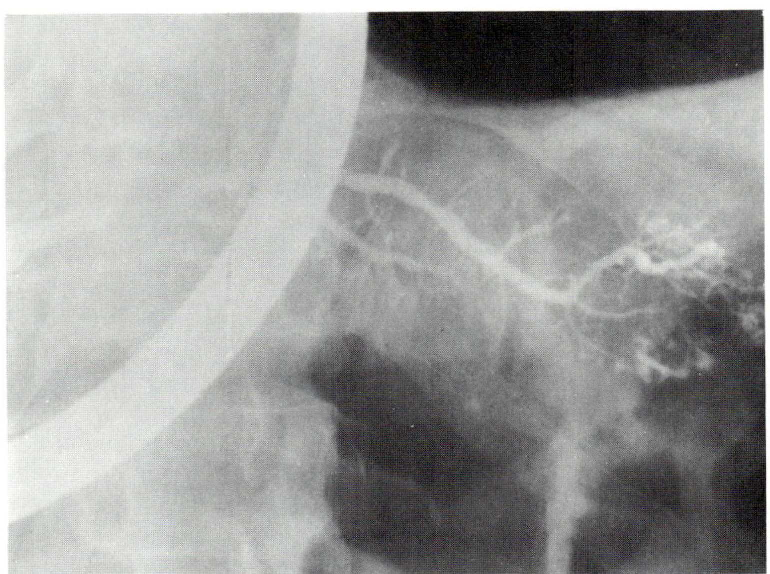

Figure 6-18.   Dilation of lateral branches in the tail of the pancreas resulting from pancreatitis.

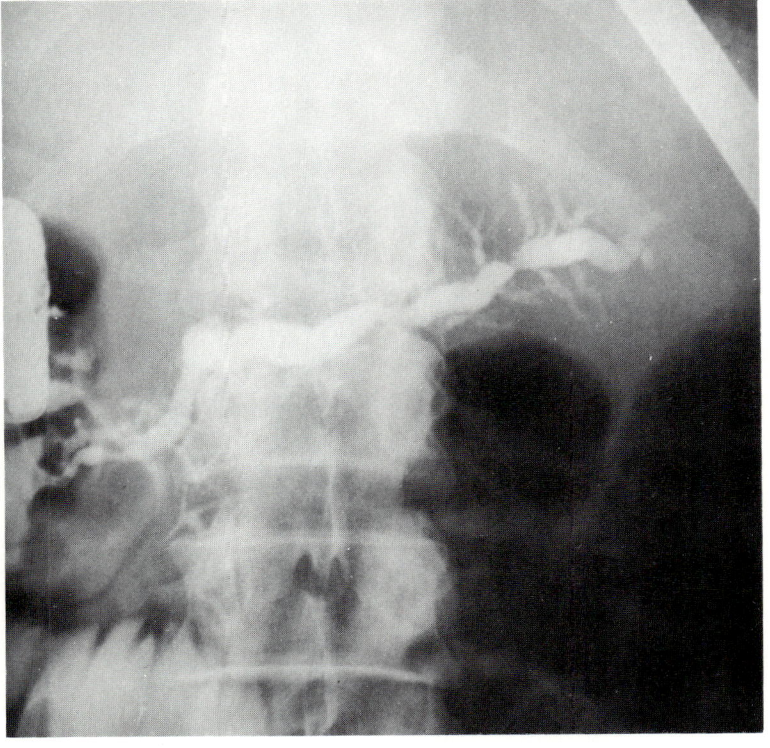

Figure 6-19.   Dilation and narrowing of the main pancreatic duct. This beading effect is diagnostic of moderately advanced chronic pancreatitis. The lateral branches are also widened.

occur in the main and branch ducts (see Fig. 6-20). Solitary or multiple stenosis, or complete obstruction may develop in the main pancreatic duct. Single or multiple cysts may form in the branch ducts. Stones may aggregate in the main duct system (see Fig. 6-21) and side branches; and a deposit of calcium may build up in the parenchyma.

Short areas of narrowing in the pancreatic duct are common, but solitary stricture longer than 1 cm is unusual, and would favor the presence of malignancy-complicating chronic pancreatitis. Obstruction of the pancreatic duct caused by malignancy may produce changes similar to chronic pancreatitis.

PSEUDOCYST.   Pancreatic pseudocyst was found in 60 patients. Pancreatic pseudocyst may be diagnosed unequivocally if the cystic cavity is filled by injection of contrast medium. If the cyst does not fill, obstruction of or a mass effect on the pancreatic duct could be caused by a cyst. Pseudocyst of significant size usually occurs in glands with moderate or advanced ductal changes (see Figs. 6-5 and 6-22). Not all pseudocysts will fill immediately by retrograde injection, and some may fill late after the ductal system has been opacified completely (see Fig. 6-23). Infection is a possible complication in cases where the cyst is filled and does not drain. The usual practice in performing ERCP is to

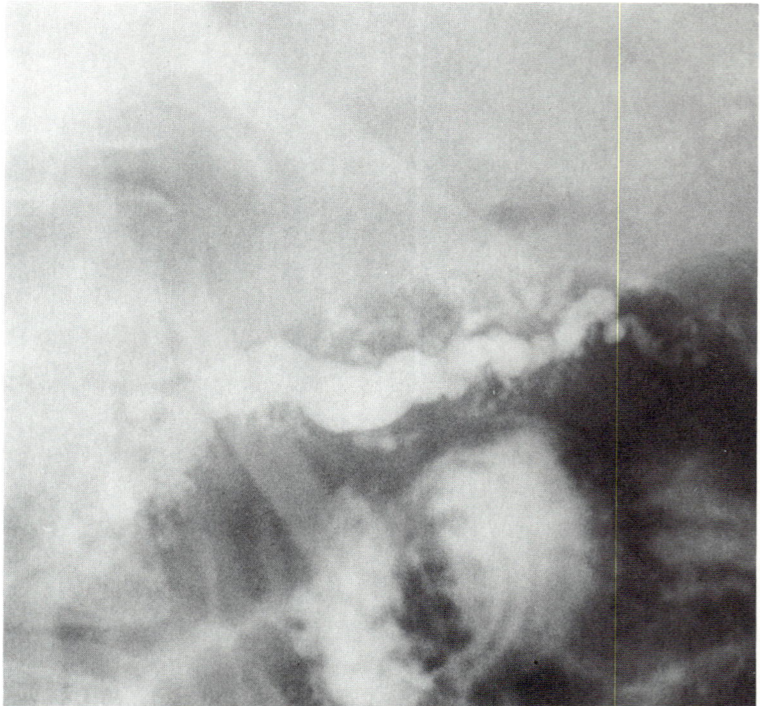

Figure 6-20.   Marked dilation of the pancreatic duct. The lateral branches are cystic. This is characteristic of advanced chronic pancreatitis.

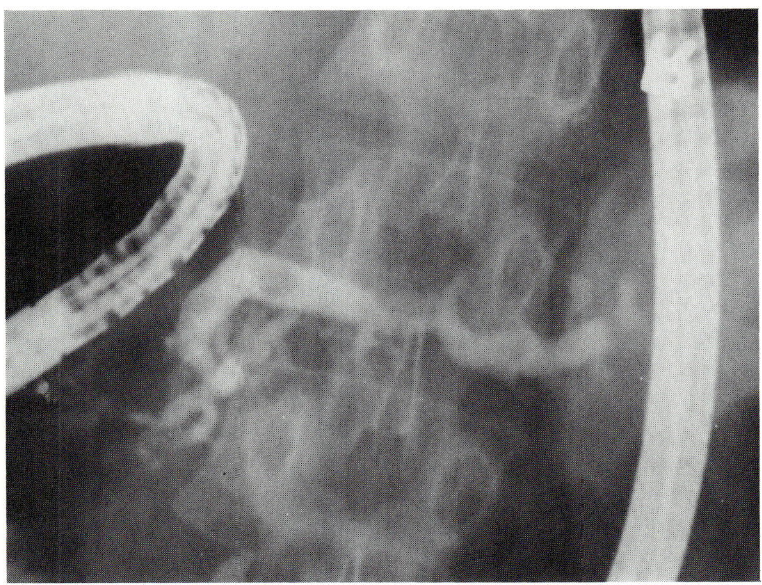

Figure 6-21.   Stones in a dilated pancreatic duct.

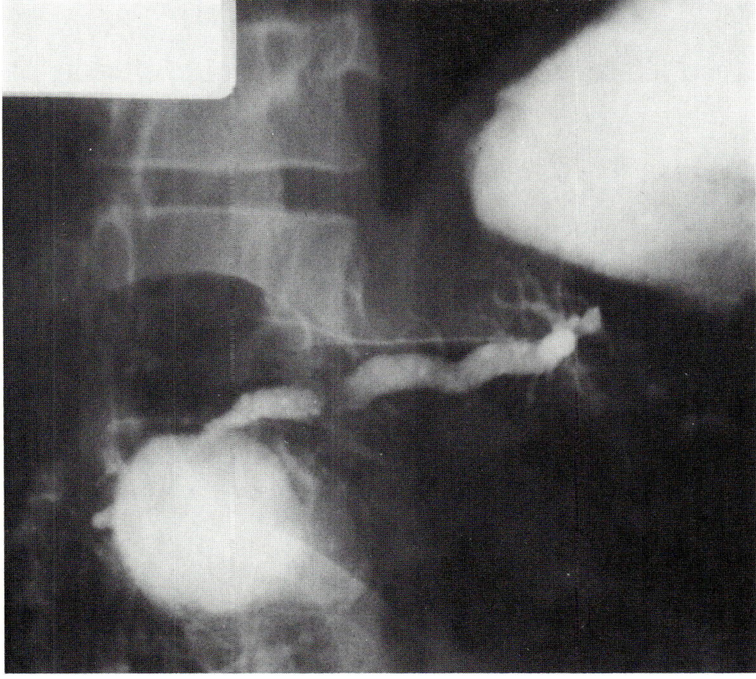

Figure 6-22.   Large pseudocyst of the head of the pancreas. The dense collection of contrast in the right upper corner of the picture is in the fundus of the stomach.

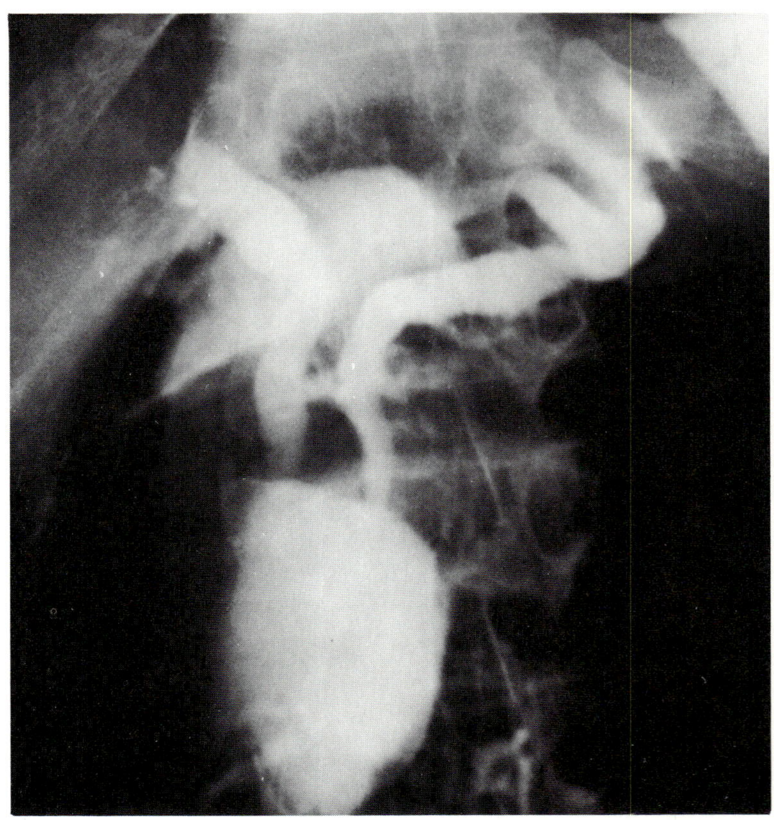

Figure 6-23.   A large pseudocyst has been filled in the head pancreas. This occurred after the initial filling of the pancreatic duct. (From C. Sugawa and A.J. Walt, Endoscopic retrograde pancreatography in the surgery of pancreatic pseudocysts. Surgery 86: 642, 1979. Reprinted courtesy of the C.V. Mosby Company.)

discontinue the injection of contrast material when the cyst is fluoro-scopically identified. In our experience, ERCP has not been responsible for pancreatic abscess when surgical drainage of the opacified cyst is accomplished within 24 hours of the study.

Pancreatography has been useful in differentiating a fistula from a pancreatic pseudocyst in other organs such as the stomach and colon (see Fig. 6-24). A leaking pseudocyst or a direct ductal leak into the peritoneal cavity, causing pancreatic ascites, has been dramatically demonstrated by ERCP.

Pancreatography has also been useful in evaluating the patency of a pancreatic enteric drainage procedure, or the condition of the pancreas after partial pancreatectomy or drainage of a pseudocyst (see Fig. 6-25).

CARCINOMA.   Cancer of the pancreas is usually a well differentiated adenocarcinoma, and virtually always arises from the duct epithelium. A majority of cases show diagnostic changes in the main pancreatic duct, common bile duct, or both; diagnostic accuracy is very high.

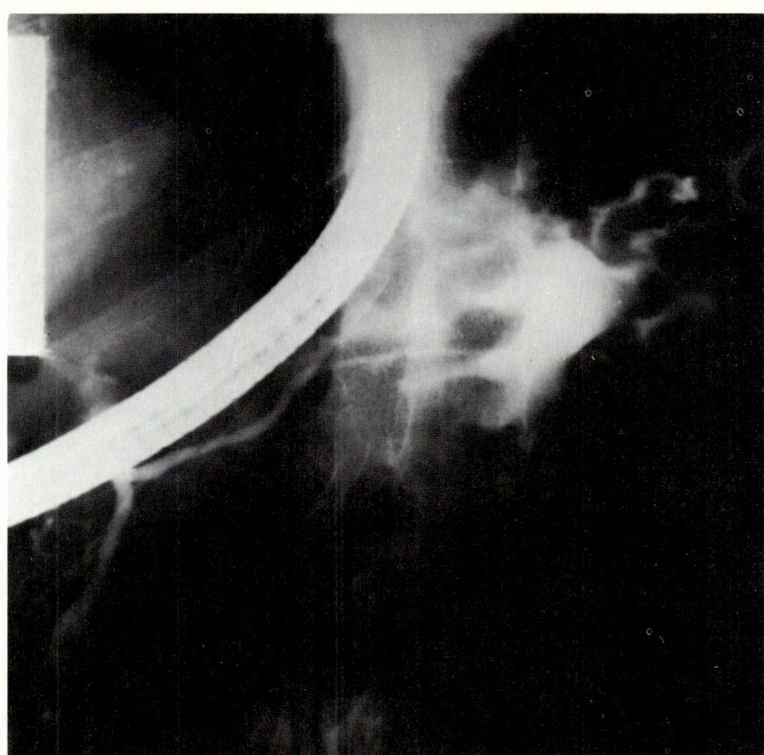

Figure 6-24. *The pseudocyst of the pancreatic tail communicates with the fundus of the stomach.*

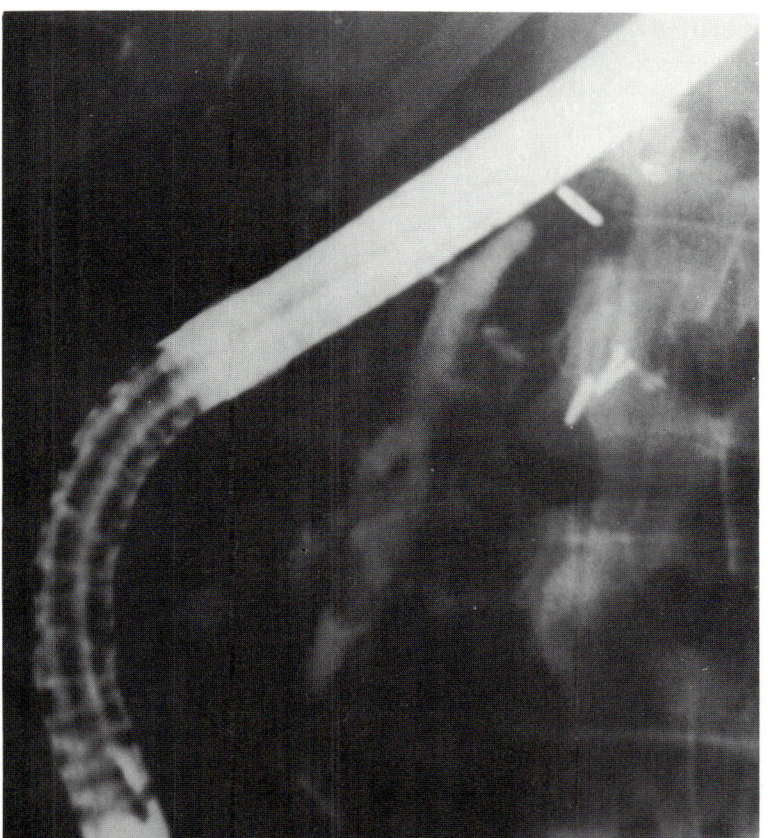

Figure 6-25. *A subtotal pancreatectomy has been performed for pseudocyst. There is a stone in the pancreatic duct remnant.*

Cancer of the pancreas with or without jaundice was found in 108 patients in our series.

Typical ductal changes for pancreatic carcinoma are

1. Irregular stenosis with or without prestenotic ectasia of the main duct (see Fig. 6-26)
2. Complete obstruction of the main duct; obstruction being abrupt or gradual (see Fig. 6-27)
3. Rigidity and marginal irregularity of the main pancreatic duct that tapers. The narrowing is extensive and branches are absent (see Fig. 6-28)
4. Ductal displacement
5. Cystic formation or a single large cavity
6. Pooling of contrast material, a result of tumor destruction
7. Stenosis of the common bile duct with irregular contour and kinking of the stenosed section

When a completely normal ductal system is demonstrated distal to the point of stenosis or obstruction, it is highly suggestive of cancer. The real diagnostic problem occurs when ERCP is done to evaluate

Figure 6-26.   Stenosis of the pancreatic duct due to carcinoma.

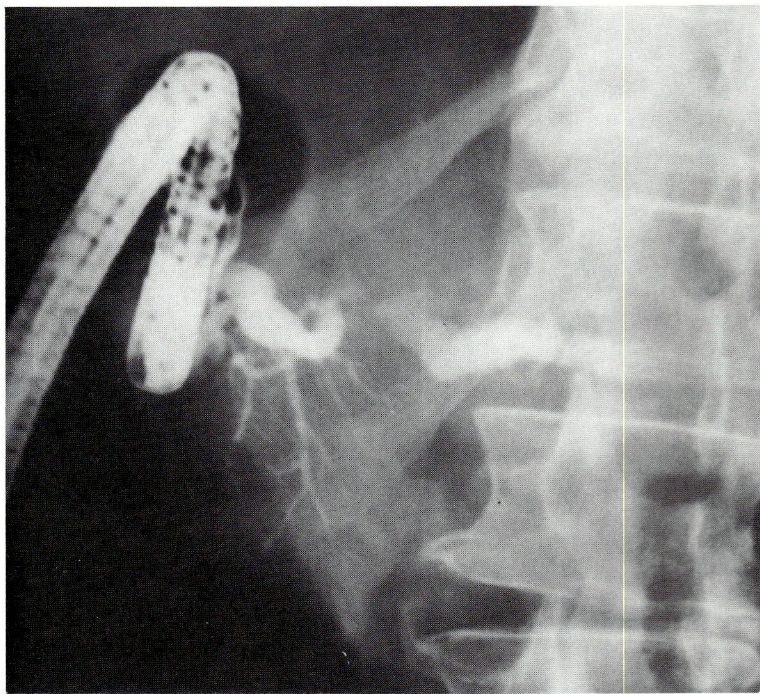

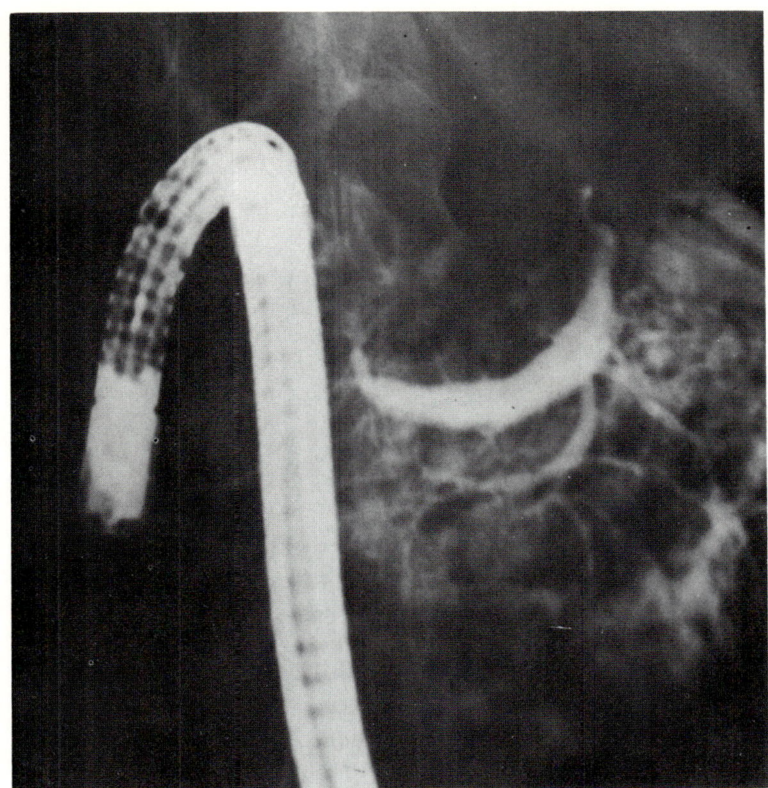

Figure 6-27.   Complete obstruction of the pancreatic duct by carcinoma.

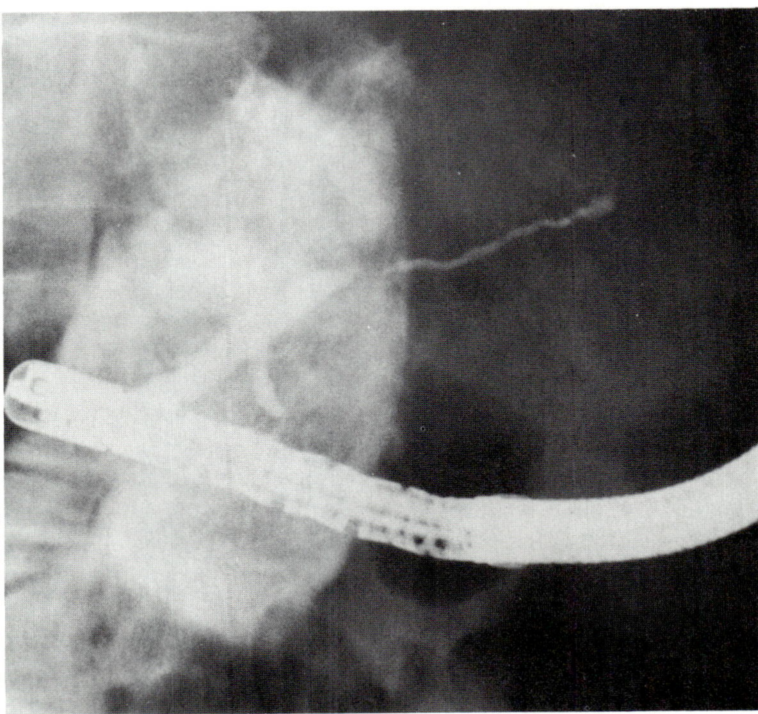

Figure 6-28.   Carcinoma of the body and tail of the pancreas.

Figure 6-29.   Arborization of the pancreatic duct within the head, characteristic of pancreas divisum. The common bile duct is seen above and below the endoscope.

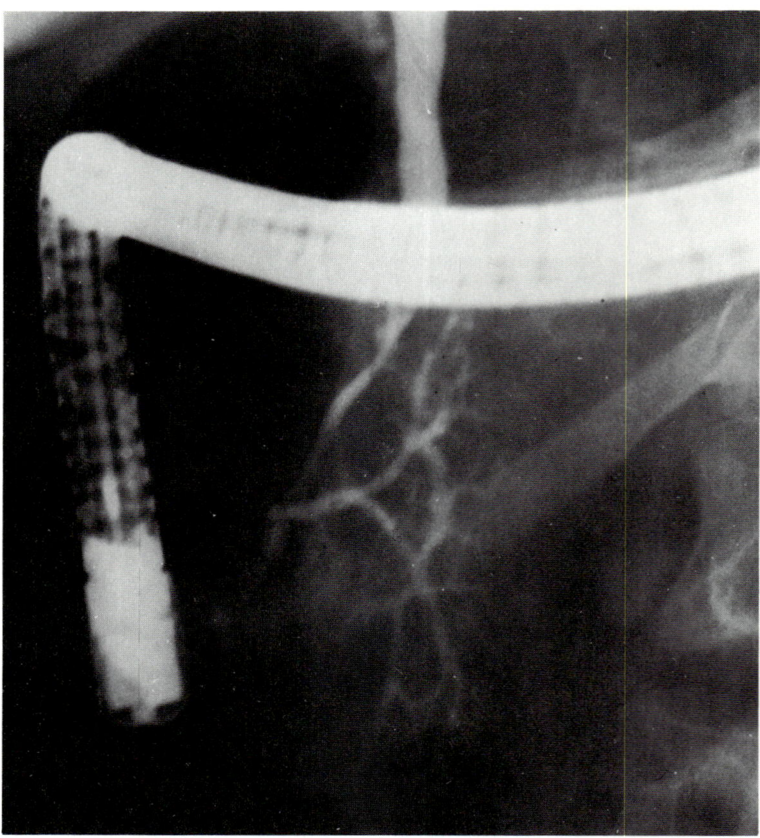

the patient with chronic pancreatitis, and a long stricture or obstruction is found. Other diagnostic modes such as ultrasonography may be invoked, but frequently, only surgical exploration will settle these difficult cases.

PANCREAS DIVISUM.   The most important variation of ductal anatomy is failure of fusion of the two embryonic duct systems with complete separation into a dorsal and ventral gland called pancreas divisum. This variant is encountered in about 3 to 4 percent of cases by ERCP. Our series includes eight cases.

In pancreas divisum, the duct of Wirsung arises from the major papilla and terminates within 5 to 7 cm (see Fig. 6-29). The duct is recognized by its small caliber. Its arborizing patterns should not be confused with an obstructed main pancreatic duct. Ductal changes due to pancreatitis can occur either in the dorsal anlage (Santorini's duct) or ventral anlage (Wirsung's duct), and methods of surgical treatment differ depending on the affected area.

SELECTED READINGS

Anacker, H., Weiss, H.D., and Kramann, B. Endoscopic Retrograde Pancreato-Cholangiography. Berlin: Springer-Verlag, 1977.

Kawanishi, H., Sell, J.E., and Pollard, H.M. Combined endoscopic pancreatic fluid collection and retrograde pancreatography in the diagnosis of pancreatic cancer and chronic pancreatitis. *Gastrointest. Endosc.* 22:82, 1975.

McGune, W.S., Shorb, P.E., and Moscovitz, H. Endoscopic cannulation of the ampulla of Vater: A preliminary report. *Ann. Surg.* 167:752, 1968.

Nebel, O.T., et al. Complications associated with endoscopic retrograde pancreatography. Results of the 1974 ASGE survey. *Gastrointest. Endosc.* 22:34, 1975.

Oi, I. Fiberduodenoscopy and endoscopic pancreatocholangiography. *Gastrointest. Endosc.* 17:59, 1970.

Sankaran, S., Sugawa C., and Walt, A.J. Value of endoscopic retrograde pancreatography in pancreatic ascites. *Surg. Gynecol. Obstet.* 148:185, 1979.

Sivak, M.V., and Sullivan, B.H. Endoscopic retrograde pancreatography. Analysis of the normal pancreatogram. *Am. J. Dig. Dis.* 21:263, 1976.

Silvis, S.E., Rohrmann, C.A., and Vennes, J.A. Diagnostic accuracy of endoscopic retrograde cholangiopancreatography in hepatic, biliary and pancreatic malignancy. *Ann. Intern. Med.* 84:438, 1976.

Silvis, S.E., Rohrmann, C.A., and Vennes, J.A. Diagnostic criteria for the evaluation of the endoscopic pancreatogram. *Gastrointest. Endosc.* 20:51, 1973.

Stewart, E.T., Dennes, J.A., and Greenen, J.E. Atlas of Endoscopic Retrograde Cholangio-Pancreatography. St. Louis: Mosby, 1977.

Sugawa, C., et al. Peroral endoscopic cholangiography and pancreatography. The surgeon's helper. *Arch. Surg.* 108:231, 1974.

Sugawa, C., et al. Pancreatic pseudocyst communicating with the stomach demonstrated by retrograde pancreatography. *Arch. Surg.* 112:1050, 1977.

Sugawa, C., and Walt, A.J. Endoscopic retrograde pancreatography in the surgery of pancreatic pseudocysts. *Surgery* 86:639, 1979.

Zimmon, D.S. Endoscopic diagnosis and management of biliary and pancreatic disease. *Curr. Probl. Surg.* 16(3):1979.

Zonca, M.C., Schuman, B.M., and Wong, K.H. The diagnosis of cancer of the biliary tract and pancreas by endoscopic retrograde cannulation. *Gastrointest. Endosc.* 21:129, 1975.

CHAPTER 7

COLONOSCOPY

Colonoscopy has become such an important diagnostic tool in the management of colonic disease that it would be difficult now for physicians concerned with diseases of the large colon to practice without it. Here is an instrument that probes every recess of the colon, allowing direct evaluation of its mucosal surface as well as documentation by photography or direct biopsy. Although the great impetus for the development of colonoscopy occurred in the 1970s, clinical experimentation with fiberoptic endoscopy for examination of the sigmoid colon was begun 10 years earlier. It was several years before the "ugly duckling" of the early prototype model would turn into a beautiful swan. An early model was just 60 cm long with a somewhat stiff and unwieldy shaft, and a tip that was only bidirectional. It was through the perseverance of Overholt and others who worked to improve its design and develop techniques for easier intubation that colonoscopy achieved its important place in the gastrointestinal diagnostic armamentarium.

In 1969, landmark papers by Overholt and Fox described a successful technique for fiberoptic colonoscopy. Wolff and Shinya, using fluoroscopy with an image intensifier, developed a large patient experience and a technique that permitted examination of the colon, and into the ileocecal valve. The manufacturers, scenting a real breakthrough in endoscopy, produced one model after another to match the skills of the growing number of enthusiastic colonoscopists. In 1971, Wolff and Shinya established colonoscopy as a standard diagnostic procedure for colonic disease by publication of their paper "Colonofiberscopy". Other endoscopists from the United States, Europe, and Japan soon reported extensive experience with the fiberoptic colonoscope. Wolff and Shinya then went on to design a snare cautery wire for the removal of colonic polyps. This pioneering work led to the virtual elimination of colotomy or colectomy for the removal of colonic polyps in any hospital where there was a skilled colonoscopist. There is no question that the 1970s were the decade of colonoscopy; this was brought about by physicians from all over the world, giving us a splendid example of scientific attainments possible through international communication and cooperation.

INSTRUMENTS AND ACCESSORIES

It is pointless to describe any particular instrument for colonoscopy. The colonoscopes are available in lengths ranging from 60 cm for the new fiberoptic sigmoidoscopes to 187 cm for the long bundle colonoscopes. New model numbers appear at frequent intervals from the manufacturing centers of the American Cystoscope Makers, Inc. (ACMI), the Olympus Optical Company, and Fujinon Company. Therefore, we will describe an ideal colonoscope that incorporates the features necessary for complete diagnostic evaluation of the colon and for therapeutic maneuvers.

The colonoscope should be 150 cm long if reasonable success in reaching the cecum is to be achieved. The colonoscopist should be trained to do a total colonoscopy just as the radiologist is trained to examine the entire colon by barium enema. A shorter colonoscope may be used at a subsequent examination to recheck a specific area, but we believe that the initial examination of the colon should be a complete one if possible. The distal tip of the colonoscope should be so controlled that it can be moved circumferentially with an arc of 120 degrees or more. The shaft of the instrument should be flexible throughout its length. The head of the scope should be designed to be grasped by the left hand, so that the fingers of the left hand can reach over to move the controls. The left hand should also be able to control air insufflation and water irrigation as well as suction. The authors believe the two-channel biopsy-suction instrument offers important advantages, but a one-channel instrument is usually sufficient to perform all necessary colonoscopic maneuvers. The two-channel instrument, however, makes possible some polypectomies that might otherwise be challenging, frustrating, and time-consuming procedures (see Fig. 7-1). In addition, there must be access for CO_2 insufflation for those colonoscopists who still fear explosion despite adequate cleansing and air insufflation of the colon.

The left hand, therefore, plays the counterpoint to the activities of the right hand. The left hand manipulates the control for direction of the tip, fingers the valves for water irrigation of the lens, suction, and air insufflation, and supports the head of the instrument. Thus the right hand is free to carry on the main procedure, which is to direct the colonoscope through frequently tortuous loops, turns, and angulations (see Fig. 7-2).

Biopsy forceps are interchangeable from one instrument to another, and any particular model of biopsy forceps can be purchased separately to use with any colonoscope. Cytology brushes are available but have little practical use in colonoscopy. Plastic catheters can be passed down the channel for irrigation with a Water Pik unit. Catheters enclosing snares, of course, can also be passed down the biopsy channels. Unfortunately, viewing attachments for teaching purposes are not interchangeable from one manufacturer to another. It is generally possible to get adapters so that any camera can be put on any instrument.

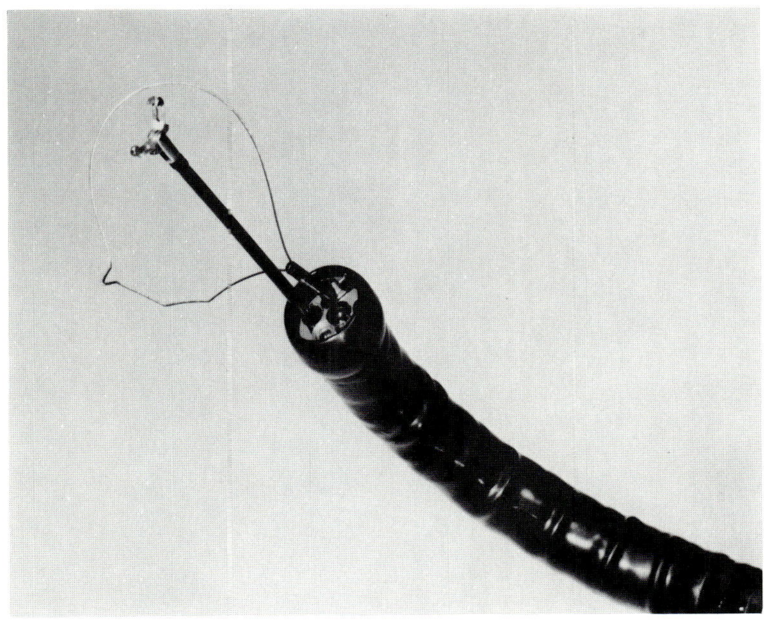

Figure 7-1.   The Olympus two-channel TCF. The biopsy forceps protrudes from one channel, and the polypectomy snare from the other.

Adapters for closed-circuit television are also available, but TV production requires considerable financial outlay.

The most important and essential accessory is, of course, the light source. The number of models of light sources do not approach the number of colonoscopic models, but there is nevertheless a wide choice. The manufacturer will sell an adaptor that will attach the colonoscope to any light source, but one must remember that an adaptor will generally reduce the amount of light available. It is most important that adequate light is available for colonoscopic examination, and the best light source available that is affordable should be purchased. It is desirable that the light source have the capability for color photography, movies, and closed-circuit television.

INDICATIONS, CONTRAINDICATIONS, AND COMPLICATIONS

Indications

Knowing when it is appropriate to employ colonoscopy in the diagnostic evaluation of a patient is as important as knowing how to use the colonoscope. Good technique is important and often crucial for a successful study. But indications should be primary and paramount. Except for unique occasions, barium enema and sigmoidoscopy are the basic resources for diagnosis of colonic disease. Colonoscopy will

Figure 7-2.   Hand positions for the co-lonoscope.

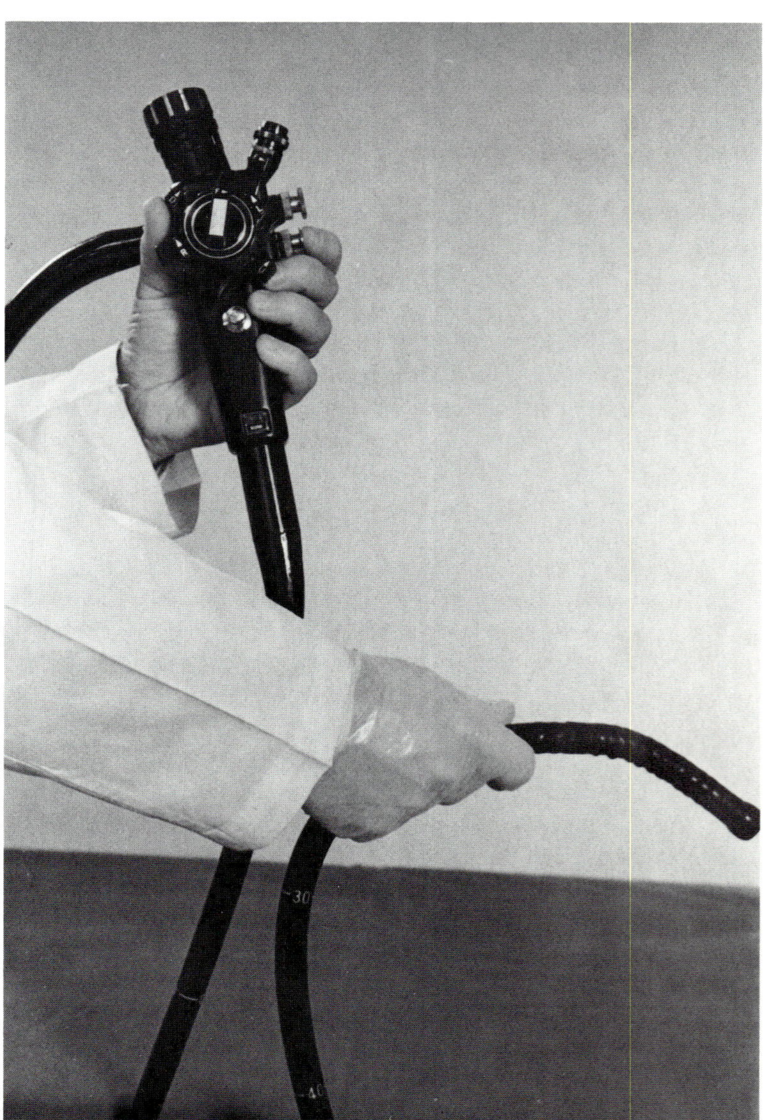

follow these studies and, therefore, the major indications are related to the barium enema examination.

When the barium study of the colon is inconclusive for polyps or for inflammatory bowel disease, colonoscopy should be invoked to settle the matter. In patients where the x-ray study is normal yet there is strong clinical reason to believe that there is underlying colonic pa-thology, colonoscopy should also be done. Where x-ray studies show conclusive evidence of a lesion, colonoscopy may be indicated to provide preoperative pathologic confirmation by biopsy, or to exclude other associated lesions that may be important in the surgical management. For unexplained bleeding without gross blood in the stool, colonoscopy would be the final diagnostic study. When there is active passage of red blood from the rectum, under some circumstances colonoscopy might be called upon as the first diagnostic study—particularly if a barium enema has been found negative in the recent past.

A polyp identified by x-ray study is an indication for colonoscopic polypectomy if this polyp is 5 mm or more in diameter. However, since the barium enema may not identify all polyps that are present, any polyp greater than 5 mm defined by barium enema would be an indication for diagnostic colonoscopy to determine the presence of other polyps or the possibility of early malignancy. Colonoscopy is indicated in those patients who have had previous polypectomy or colon resection for cancer if the routine barium enema study proves inadequate because of difficulty in bowel preparation or difficulty in interpretation of surgical changes at the site of resection. Rarely is the colonoscope used for the removal of foreign bodies from the colon. Under appropriate conditions, research studies may be carried out for the evaluation of drug therapy of chronic inflammatory bowel disease or for the evaluation of histologic changes in various disease states. In patients who have a high risk for the development of colon cancer as in ulcerative colitis, the regular use of colonoscopy, or at least of fiberoptic sigmoidoscopy, may be indicated to achieve earlier detection of malignancy.

Contraindications

Colonoscopy should not be done in any patient who has evidence of acute inflammatory disease of the colon. Thus, colonoscopy is contraindicated because of the high risk of perforation in patients with acute, ulcerative, or granulomatous colitis, acute diverticulitis, or severe colitis due to drug or irradiation therapy. In addition, patients with recent pelvic inflammatory disease or those who are pregnant should not have this procedure done, although a unique circumstance may arise to warrant the increased risk. Suspected perforation or peritonitis from any cause contraindicates the procedure. Patients who have serious cardiopulmonary disease or who have had a recent myocardial infarction are not candidates. Intraabdominal abnormalities such as an aneurysm of the iliac artery or the aorta, huge splenomegaly, a large pancreatic pseudocyst, or massive ascites are contraindications. Where contraindications of lesser importance exist such as anemia, coronary insufficiency, chronic obstructive lung disease, recent abdominal or pelvic surgery, or perianal disease, one must weigh the risks of colonoscopy against those risks of an alternative procedure, and also weigh in the balance the possible benefits of colonoscopy not obtained otherwise.

Complications

There is no doubt that fiberoptic colonoscopy represents a major advance in the diagnosis and treatment of colonic disease. The remarkable success of this procedure, however, should not blind us to the fact that there are dangers associated with colonoscopy. Many authors extolling the value of colonoscopy from their early experience glossed over or minimized the complications. Colcher, in a report to the American Society for Gastrointestinal Endoscopy surveyed 124 colonoscopists among whose patients were 45 free and 11 closed perforations as well as 54 bleeding episodes. Three deaths were related to these complications. In a later study from the Medical College of Wisconsin, 1106 colonoscopies performed by 28 physicians revealed 14 complications, or 1.2 percent of the total number of procedures. Seven out of nine perforations occurred during diagnostic procedures, but all of the bleeding episodes were a result of polypectomy. A large survey of complications from colonoscopy was compiled in 1974 by the Research Committee of the American Society for Gastrointestinal Endoscopy. A total of 24,119 colonoscopic procedures were scrutinized. Forty-nine perforations of the colon and 75 bleeding events were recorded for an incidence of 0.5 percent.

Of interest were 63 patients at Henry Ford Hospital in Detroit, who had continuous electrocardiographic monitoring before, during, and after colonoscopy. One third showed no electrocardiographic abnormalities but the remainder showed new or more electrocardiographic abnormalities. These included sinus tachycardia and bradycardia; premature ventricular, atrial, and junctional contractions; ST-T segment depression; intermittent left bundle branch block; and paroxysmal atrial tachycardia. The more serious arrhythmias occurred in patients with underlying heart disease. These findings confirm the small adverse effect on the normal cardiovascular system with colonoscopy, but it would be wise to monitor patients with underlying heart disease.

Another issue that has been raised is that of bacteremia or septicemia associated with colonoscopy. There have been conflicting reports in the literature regarding this matter. Although some authors have identified bacteremia in association with colonoscopy, septicemia or endocarditis has never been reported. Bacteremia is transient if it does occur, and is of doubtful significance. Norfleet studied a group of patients in whom no bacteremia was detected and this work has been confirmed by one of the authors [B.M.S.]. It would appear that prophylactic antibiotics are not required in patients undergoing colonoscopy, except in the presence of a cardiac valve prosthesis.

HISTORY AND PHYSICAL EXAMINATION

It is mandatory that the colonoscopist be familiar with the patient's medical history and physical examination. A history of cardiovascular disease in the past does not contraindicate the procedure but certainly should alert the physician to the possible effects on cardiac rhythm by vago-vagal reflexes. In patients with a history of cardiac arrhythmia, cardiac monitoring is essential. The risk of bacterial endocarditis in patients with valvular disease of the heart seems to be remote and our own experience with 26 patients who had negative multiple blood cultures during colonoscopy confirms this impression. Patients with hypertension should have blood pressure surveillance during the procedure. A history of a clotting disorder demands a thorough evaluation prior to polypectomy. Any known allergic reaction to drugs should be recounted to members of the team.

Physical findings such as an enlarged liver or enlarged spleen should be confirmed by the colonoscopist and evaluated from the point of hepatosplenomegaly contributing to the likelihood of a complication. In elderly patients, the examination should include a careful search for an aneurysm of the abdominal aorta. In view of the considerable insufflation of the colon or small bowel that might occur in the course of colonoscopy, the examiner should be alert for the presence of hernias; these may be inguinal, ventral, incisional, or hiatal. Patients with cirrhosis of the liver offer special problems with regard to coagulation, ascites, and response to intravenous ataractic and analgesic agents. Increased abdominal pressure may lead to distention of esophageal varices and may theoretically bring about a complication of bleeding, rather remote from the actual colonoscopic procedure. In other words, a colonoscopist with tunnel vision who does not also see his patient as a repository of a medical history could find himself in serious trouble.

A review of all laboratory data should be made prior to the endoscopy. The blood count should be within an acceptable range. Renal or hepatic laboratory abnormalities should be evaluated. Coagulation should be studied by a prothrombin time, partial thromboplastin time, and platelet count prior to any possible polypectomy. A current electrocardiogram should be in the record to serve as a baseline reference should there be any untoward cardiovascular reaction.

The barium enema film should be carefully reviewed before the procedure so that the colonoscopist can familiarize himself with the anatomy of the patient's colon. Careful attention must be given to the sigmoid loop, so that the examiner has some idea of what may be required to negotiate the sigmoid colon. The extent of diverticulosis of the colon should be carefully noted. The heights to which the splenic flexure might reach as well as the depths to which the midtransverse colon may drop should not escape notice. Any redundant loops at the flexures should be observed. The redundancy of the cecum and its position in the abdomen should be noted. It is wise to have a game plan prior to colonoscopy. From the x-ray findings, it is often possible to anticipate where the difficulties of intubation may lie, and therefore be prepared to handle these technical challenges. Representative films of the barium enema examination should be displayed throughout the whole procedure for reference.

PATIENT PREPARATION
Patient Preparation
The patient should be informed of the nature of the procedure and of its possible complications. A complete disclosure that is unduly and unnecessarily vivid may create such anxiety, however, that the colonoscopy examination itself is compromised. The endoscopist must judge how much and how explicit a description to give. At a minimum, the patient should know that there will be discomfort associated with the procedure but that intravenous sedation will be given to allay tension and reduce pain. The patient must also be made aware of the fact of life that a complication is possible even under the best of circumstances. Therefore, an intimation or a discourse (depending on the physician's assessment of the patient's desire to know) on the risk of bowel wall injury or, in the case of polypectomy, of bleeding must be given. A medical colonoscopist should inform the patient that surgical consultation and perhaps operation may be necessary should a serious complication ensue. A surgical endoscopist, of course, has the advantage of not requiring an intermediary to manage a complication.

Adequate cleansing of the bowel is essential for a safe and thorough examination of the colon. This requires considerable cooperation from the patient who must understand the importance of a thorough bowel preparation. For a diagnostic procedure, it is usually adequate to be on a clear liquid diet for 24 hours prior to the study. The afternoon before the procedure, 10 ounces of citrate of magnesia may be taken by mouth or 3 tablets of Dulcolax may be adequate in patients who are not ordinarily constipated. Elderly or constipated patients may require a longer or more intensive preparation. The night before and the morning of the procedure a cleansing tap water or saline enema should be given. It may require 1 to 3 liters to do this. Diagnostic colonoscopies are usually outpatient procedures, and the patient should be encouraged to drink clear liquids the day of the procedure as well as the day before. Patients who have had experience with other gastrointestinal procedures assume that nothing may be taken by mouth 12 hours before the examination, and despite word to the contrary will present themselves for colonoscopy in a dehydrated and somewhat debilitated condition.

When a polypectomy is planned, the clear liquid diet should be extended to 48 hours before the procedure, but otherwise no change is necessary in preparation. In the authors' experience, this preparation has permitted colonoscopy in almost all patients. Where room air insufflation is used, there can be no compromise regarding the thoroughness of the preparation for polypectomy.

It is obvious that not all patients can tolerate this type of thorough cleansing. Patients with inflammatory bowel disease who are considered candidates for colonoscopy may tolerate only a mild laxative and enema. Elderly patients may require longer periods of clear liquid and the diet may have to be supplemented with elemental liquid feedings. Surprisingly, geriatric patients after vigorous bowel preparation do not show significant alteration of electrolyte balance as long as their renal status is reasonably well preserved, although there may be some weight loss due to dehydration.

Premedication

It is the practice of the authors not to give intramuscular medication prior to the procedure for outpatients who may arrive shortly before the time of the study. As other authors have noted, intravenous medication just before the procedure, and titrated to the patient's anxiety level and pain threshold during the procedure, works out best. In all outpatients a butterfly needle is inserted and the catheter is kept open with a syringe of saline. Diazepam (2.5–10.0 mg) is given slowly until the patient becomes drowsy or his speech becomes slurred. The vein is then flushed with the saline syringe. Following the insertion of the colonoscope and the distention of the bowel, meperidine (25–50 mg) or diazepam (5–20 mg) may be given during the procedure should the patient show a low tolerance for this type of manipulation. In general, anticholinergic drugs are avoided because of the tendency of the relaxed bowel to become overdistended, and because with patients in the geriatric age group, the anticholinergic drugs may have adverse cardiac, eye, or urinary bladder consequences. However, some patients show a vagal reaction to torsion of the mesentery and develop a rather pronounced bradycardia; in these circumstances it is wise to give atropine (0.4 mg) intravenously. Occasionally, intravenous glucagon (0.5–1.0 mg) will be useful to induce temporary reduction of bowel motility, particularly at the time of polypectomy. It is important to realize that there can be no standard dosage for achieving sedation. Careful monitoring of the patient during intravenous titration will permit the patient to undergo colonoscopy in reasonable comfort and, following the procedure, to become alert in a short time, sometimes with amnesia of the colonoscopic event.

TECHNIQUE OF COLONOSCOPY

Room

The examining room for colonoscopy should be adequate in size, primarily so that a table can fit with sufficient room for people to circulate about it. A cart for the light source is required as well as for electrocoagulation equipment (Fig. 2-7). It is helpful for the trainee to learn colonoscopy by having the patient on a fluoroscopic tilt-table. Although the experienced colonoscopist can get along without fluoroscopy, it is desirable to have ready access to a fluoroscopy table. There should be an emergency kit containing the usual resuscitative drugs in the room and oxygen should be on hand as well as an airway and ambu bag. No patient should have colonoscopy or, for that matter, any gastrointestinal endoscopy without adequate resuscitative equipment available and ready for use by trained personnel.

There is no "royal road" that everyone must follow for a successful and safe colonoscopy. Excellent differing techniques have been developed by experienced colonoscopists. To provide a description of the variety of methods would only confuse the beginners. The authors have evolved a technique influenced by the writings and vivid presentations of Waye and of Williams.

Position of the Patient and Examination Technique

The patient lies on his left side supporting his lower body on the right knee, which has been put across the left leg (see Fig. 7-3). The examiner gloves his right hand, and lubricates the anus and perianal skin with an anesthetic jelly. A digital examination is carried out to be sure that the rectum is free of solid material, and to dilate the anal sphincter. The tip of the colonoscope is also lubricated and with the gloved hand, the index finger gently insinuates the tip of the colonoscope into the rectal vault. Should there be any resistance on the insertion of the colonoscope, this can be eliminated by having the patient gently bear down (see Fig. 7-4).

There are four obstacles that must be hurdled to accomplish a complete colonoscopy. For the beginner, the most difficult by far is the intubation of the sigmoid colon and sigmoid–descending colon junction. The next challenge is the negotiation of the splenic flexure, and the third troublesome area is the hepatic flexure. Finally, establishing that

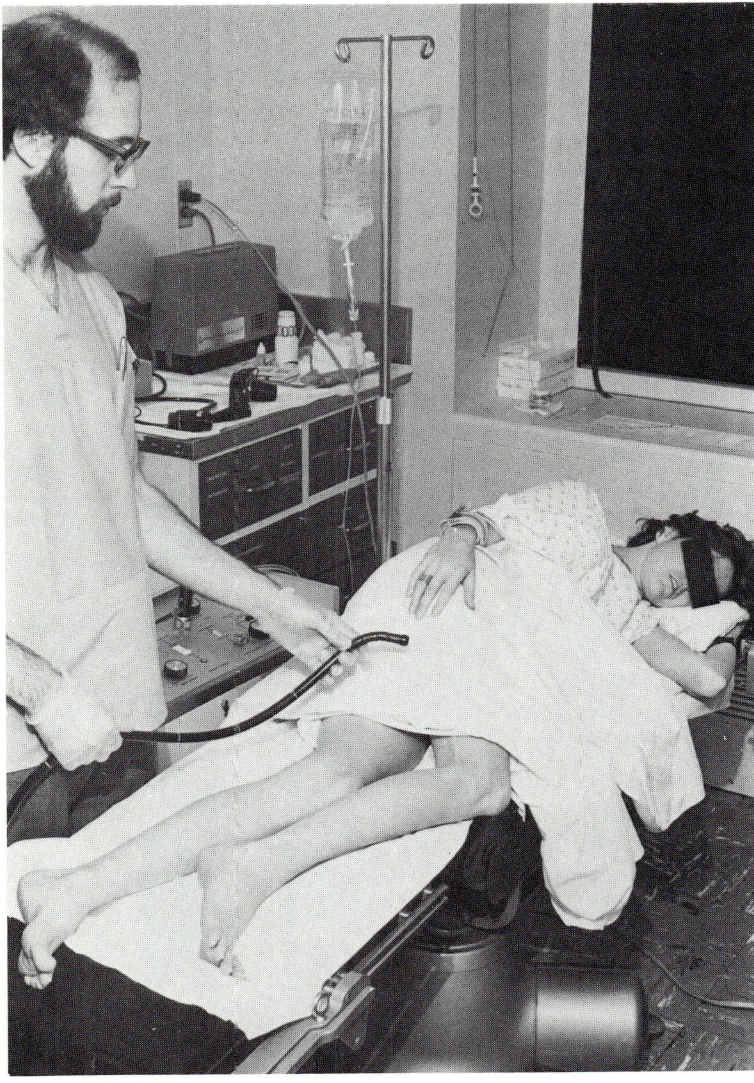

Figure 7-3.   Standard left lateral decubitus position for the patient prior to beginning colonoscopy.

the tip of the cecum has been reached may be worrisome. Of course, intubating the ileocecal valve requires considerable perseverance and dexterity, but is not usually considered an essential part of the examination.

Much has been written about achieving a successful passage of the sigmoid colon. As experience is gained, more and more emphasis is placed on passing the colonoscope only when the lumen is open, or can be anticipated behind a fold. The slide-by technique endorsed early on by Overholt is risky in the hands of the neophyte, and unnecessary

Figure 7-4. *Insertion of the colonoscopic tip into the anus.*

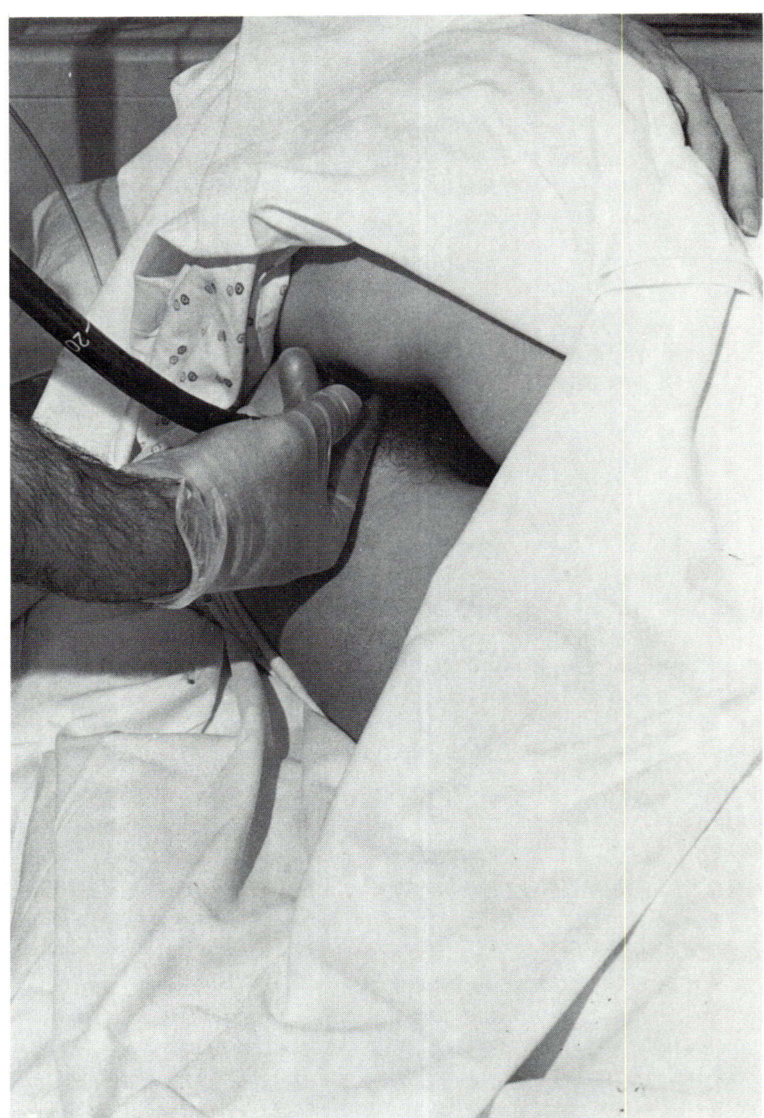

for most experienced colonoscopists. This technique involves allowing the tip of the colonoscope to advance by observing the mucosa to slide by and, as long as there is no indication of pressure by blanching of the mucosa or undue pain on the part of the patient, the instrument is allowed to progress by "gentle persuasion." Waye's method, based on several thousand colonoscopic examinations, consists of bringing the lumen into view by twisting the shaft of the instrument with the right hand which holds the colonoscope at the anal orifice. The left hand turns the controls for vertical leverage, with the right and left control locked in the appropriate direction. While this maneuver is being carried out, there is a constant insertion and withdrawal of the colonoscope in order to straighten out each loop, in effect pleating the bowel over the colonoscope. Perseverance with this technique will allow intubation to the splenic flexure in the majority of patients, unless there has been fixation of the sigmoid loops due to adhesions from previous surgery, or by episodes of diverticulitis.

Frequently, following intubation of the sigmoid colon as it curves gently to the left from the rectum, the instrument will be advanced but there will be no forward movement of the tip. This means that the colonoscope is pushing the distal loop of the sigmoid into a larger inverted U pattern; this can be confirmed under the fluoroscope (see Fig. 7-5A) or by simply palpating the abdomen and feeling the loop. Usually the technique of hooking the instrument by acutely bending the tip at the point where the lumen is lost and withdrawing it in a jiggling fashion will gradually straighten the loop over the colonoscope, and allow passage into the descending colon.

Another technique has been to move the patient into the supine position and rotate the colonoscope 180 degrees counterclockwise, so that the curve of the loop is in the right lower quadrant. Under the fluoroscope (and this should be done with fluoroscopic control for the safety of the patient) the colonoscope is now in the shape of the Greek letter alpha. Some endoscopists who use fluoroscopy routinely put the patient into the alpha position at the onset of the study.

It is possible for the sigmoid loop to reform as the colonoscope is advanced into the descending colon. This can be readily identified when it is realized that the colonoscope is being pushed into the bowel without a similar degree of forward progress of the tip of the instrument (see Fig. 7-5B). This again can be prevented by repeatedly withdrawing the instrument with the tip hooked into the bowel wall. Once the tip of the colonoscope is around the splenic flexure, this stabilizes the instrument sufficiently so that the loop almost always can be reduced.

For those doctors using fluoroscopy, an external stiffener can be used to prevent reformation of the loop. The stiffener must be put on beforehand over the long colonoscope; once it is determined under fluoroscopy that the sigmoid loop has been straightened, the stiffener can then be advanced into the rectum and for a distance of 20 or 30 cm into the sigmoid colon (see Fig. 7-6). The stiffener cannot be put in position if the alpha loop persists. This technique, if used at all, should only be done by colonoscopists who have become quite adept with the instrument, but when this degree of expertise is reached, the colonos-

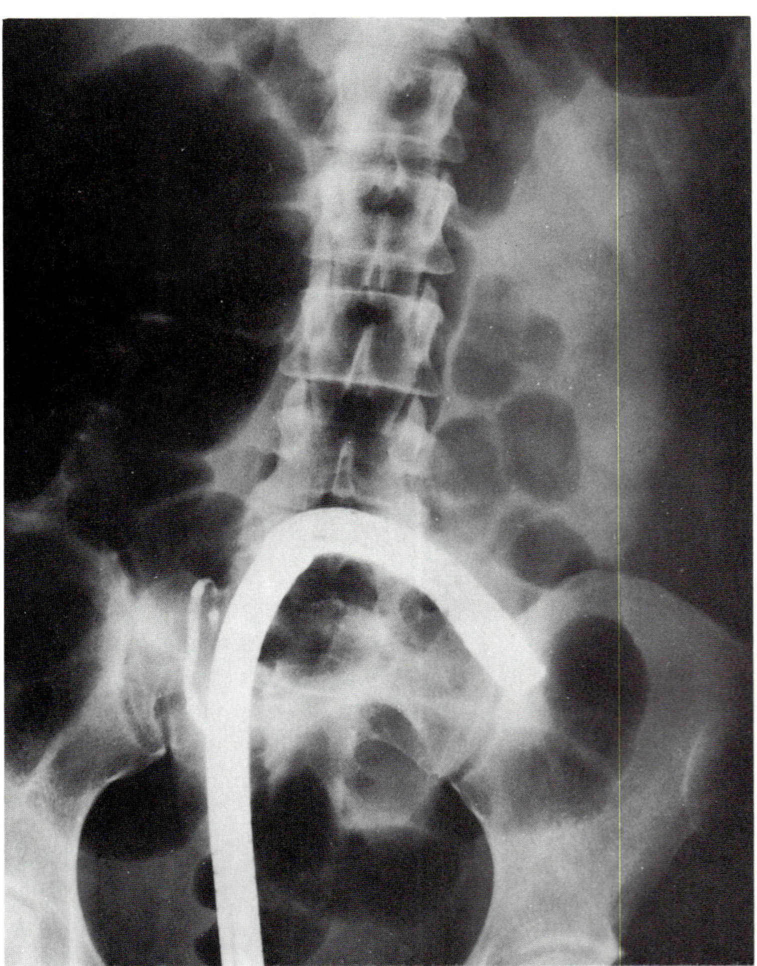

A

Figure 7-5. A. The sigmoid loop is being pushed out of the pelvis. There is barium in the appendix. B. The sigmoid loop is enlarged as the colonoscope is advanced. The loop must be reduced before further progress can be made.

copist infrequently needs the straightener. It is also possible to use an internal splint to make the colonoscope more rigid in its course through the sigmoid, and so prevent reformation of a loop as the colonoscope is moved forward. However, these devices increase the hazards for the patient and promote damage to the instrument. The wise endoscopist should consider the use of the stiffener only when safer techniques have failed.

Once safely out of the sigmoid maze, it should be easy to proceed up the descending colon to the splenic flexure. Occasionally there will be a redundant loop of the descending colon or a bowel kink that might create problems, but this can be anticipated from the barium enema

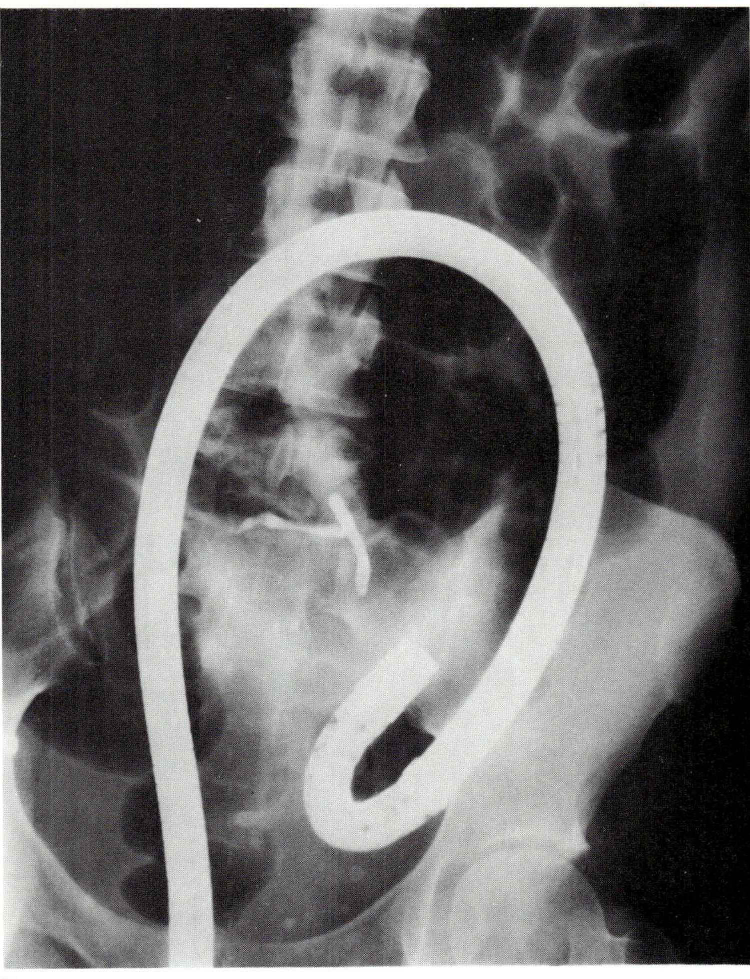

B

and usually traversed promptly. Should the lumen of the descending colon be lost, one can relocate the lumen by directing the colonoscope toward the concavity of the arc of the highlight along the ridge of a colonic fold. One can generally appreciate that the flexure has been reached by the cathedral dome appearance, and also by inspecting the abdomen for the light shining through the lower intercostal spaces (see Fig. 7-7). In a high-lying splenic flexure, the transverse colon must be entered by withdrawing the instrument somewhat, aspirating air, and directing the tip to the patient's right. By putting torsion on the instrument to enhance the tendency for the instrument to proceed to the right, the lumen of the transverse colon will be brought into view (see

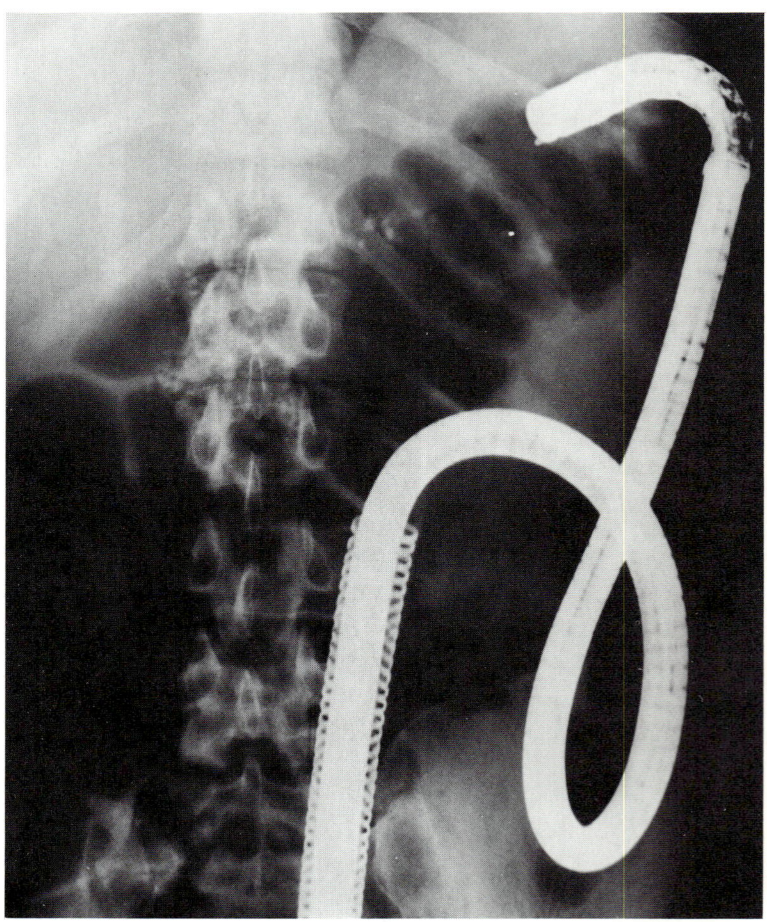

Figure 7-6. The external stiffener tube is in place.

Fig. 7-8). In the normal colon, the appearance of the lumen of the transverse colon is characteristic and unmistakable, since the three teniae coli lend a triangular appearance to the lumen.

The colonoscope will usually proceed by its own weight down the transverse colon, taking up the slack that occurred when the splenic flexure was being negotiated. From this point on there is no problem in proceeding, as the colonoscope can be kept straight by using the splenic loop as a fulcrum to reduce any loops that might have re-formed. If the transverse colon dips into the pelvis, it may be necessary to pull the scope back to straighten the colon. Arrival at the hepatic flexure can be determined by observing light shining through the abdomen in the right upper quadrant as well as by the colonoscopist reaching over and repetitively indenting the abdominal wall so that he

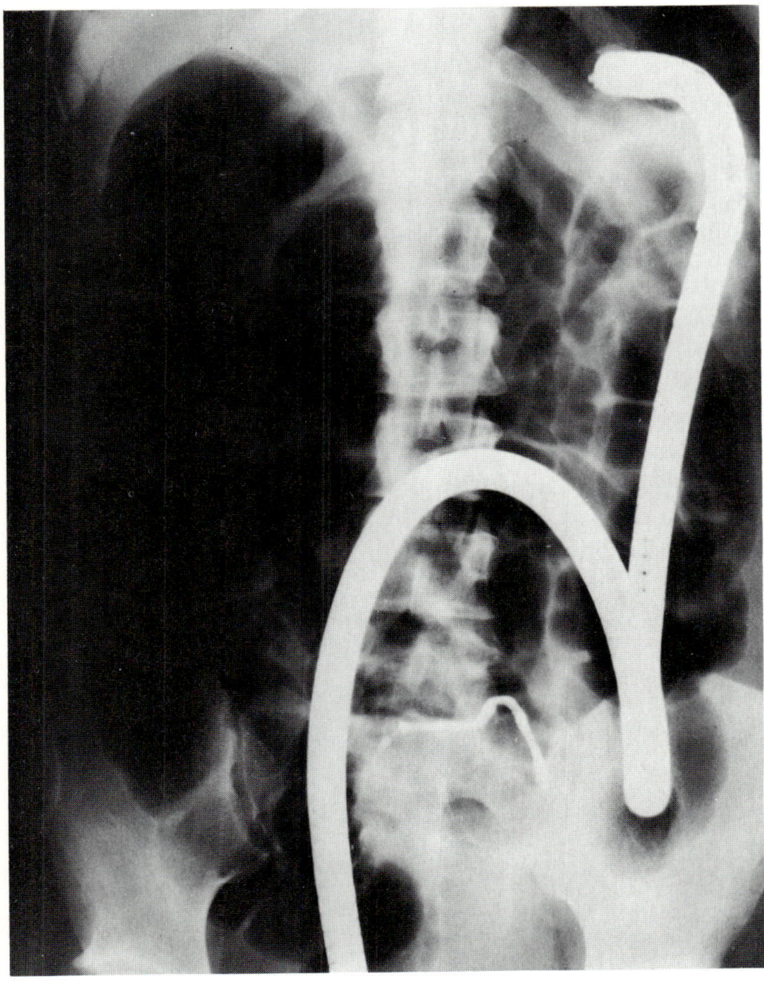

Figure 7-7.   The tip of the colonoscope is in the splenic flexure.

or she can see the transmission of the movement to the tip of the co-lonoscope (see Fig. 7-9). As in the splenic flexure, it is easier to negotiate the hepatic flexure if only the volume of air just necessary to visualize the lumen is used. Overdistention of the flexure will cause an acute angle to form at the junction of the two long segments of bowel and make it almost impossible to negotiate the flexure. Putting the patient in the supine position may assist in turning the tip into the ascending colon (see Fig. 7-10).

It is easy to get lost in the right colon. The haustra are large and the folds separating the haustra are irregular and asymmetric in distribution. If the ascending colon is overdistended, one can spend consider-able time finding his way out of one haustrum into another.

Figure 7-8.   The tip has been advanced into the transverse colon.

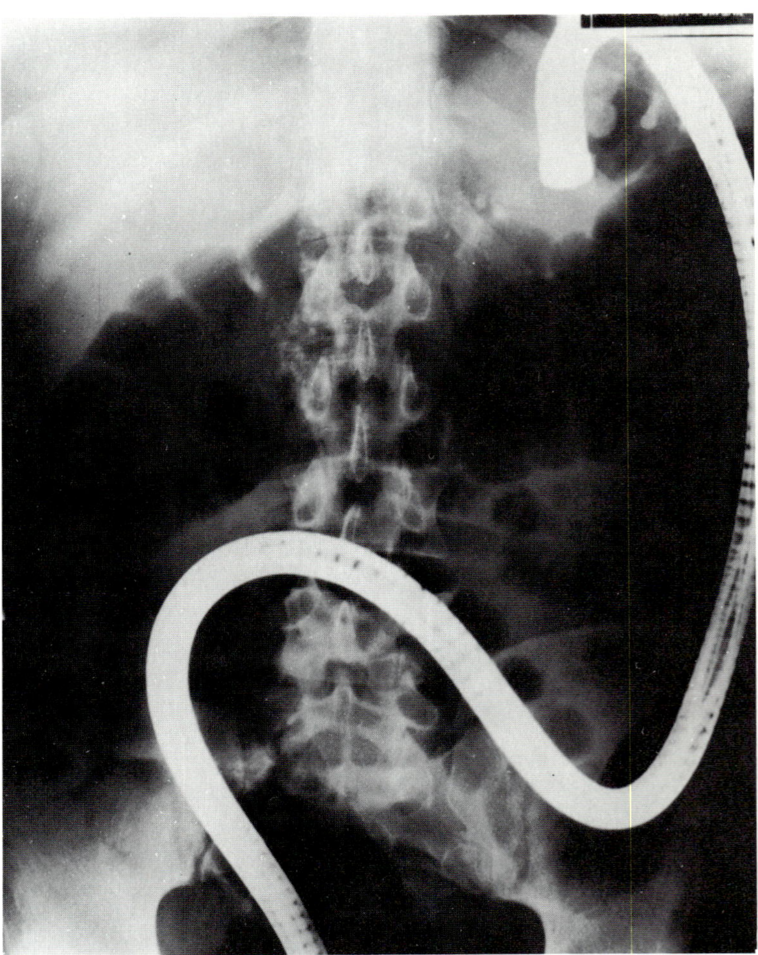

Sometimes there is uncertainty as to whether the cecum has actually been reached. Although a light may be visible in the area of the right groin, it is not necessarily the case that the full extent of the colon has been traversed. (The position of the light on the abdominal wall can be quite misleading for any segment of the colon.) The dependable but infrequently identified sign is the appendiceal os. If the ileocecal valve has been found, then intubation a few centimeters beyond should bring you to the cecum, which often has a puddle of green ileal effluent. The fold pattern of the cecum is more complex than that of the rest of the right colon and the characteristic pattern of these prominent folds is another important clue. At times, only fluoroscopy can provide assurance that the true depth has been plumbed (see Fig. 7-11).

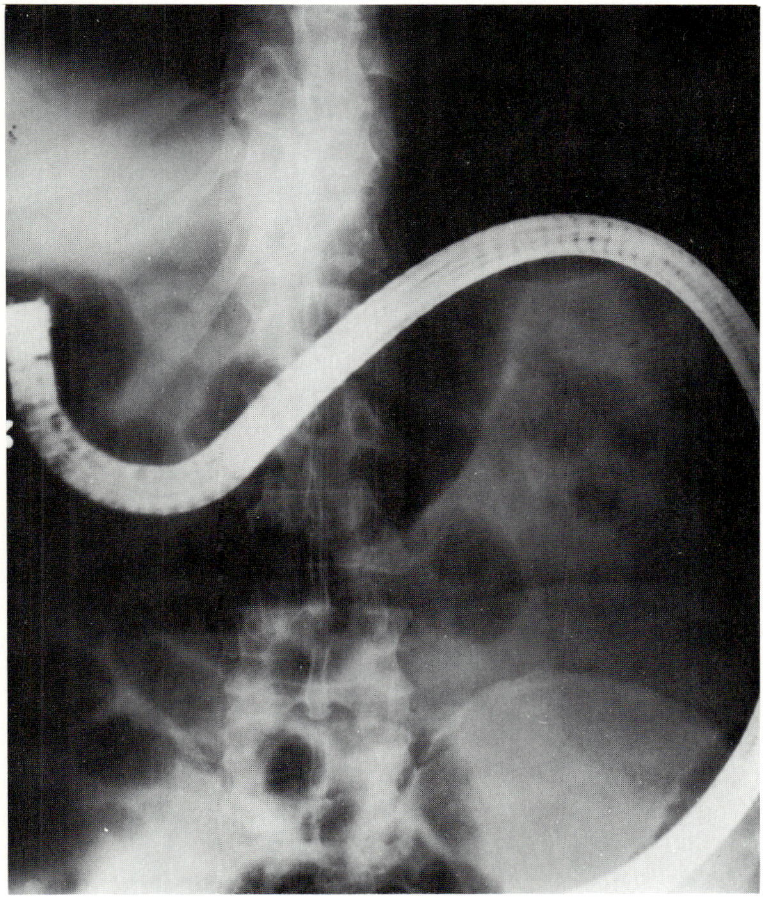

Figure 7-9.   *The tip is at the hepatic flexure.*

The ileocecal valve is sequestered among folds of the medial wall of the cecum, and usually must be sought after with diligence. The valve has a labial presentation with the larger lip generally overhanging the opening of the valve. Occasionally, the ileal contents may be seen oozing out of the stoma, and this will provide direction for intubation. It is possible to enter the ileum directly in some patients or by bending the tip of the colonoscope toward the medial wall and falling into it by chance. Intubation of the ileum, however, is best accomplished under fluoroscopic control. The ileal mucosa can be recognized by the irregular contour of its surface created by the submucosal lymphoid follicles, but this is less apparent in the older patient. Once in the ileum, one does not get too far beyond the valve because of the impedance of short loops.

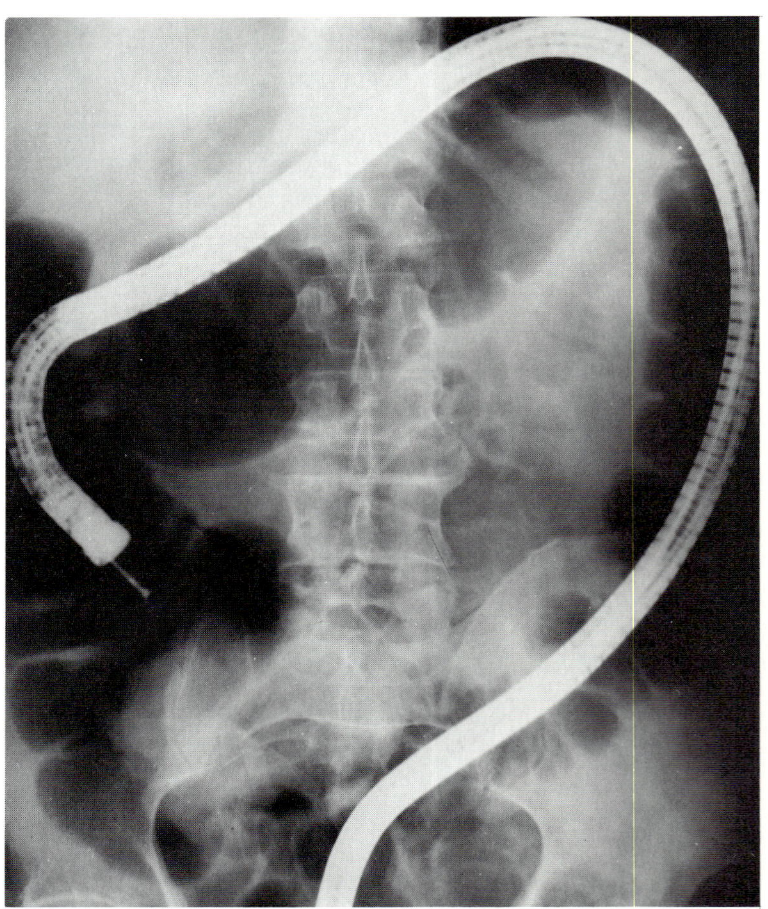

Figure 7-10. *The tip is moving into the ascending colon. A biopsy forceps is protruding into the lumen. Note that the colon has been converted into a question mark configuration.*

Duration of the Examination

How long does it take to complete a colonoscopy? Some superstars routinely reach the cecum in less than 30 minutes. But certainly those colonoscopists who are young in experience will require at least 30 minutes and usually much longer for a total colonoscopy. Many factors influence the length of time needed to complete the procedure. The tortuosity of the sigmoid loops, the position of the splenic flexure, the extent to which the transverse colon may dip into the lower abdomen, and finally the degree of redundancy of the right colon must all be contended with. In addition to the anatomic obstacles, one must also consider previous pelvic and abdominal surgery, past inflammatory reactions in the pelvis or about the sigmoid colon, the presence of hepatosplenomegaly, and perhaps most importantly, the individual sensitivity of each patient to torsion of the bowel, stretching of the

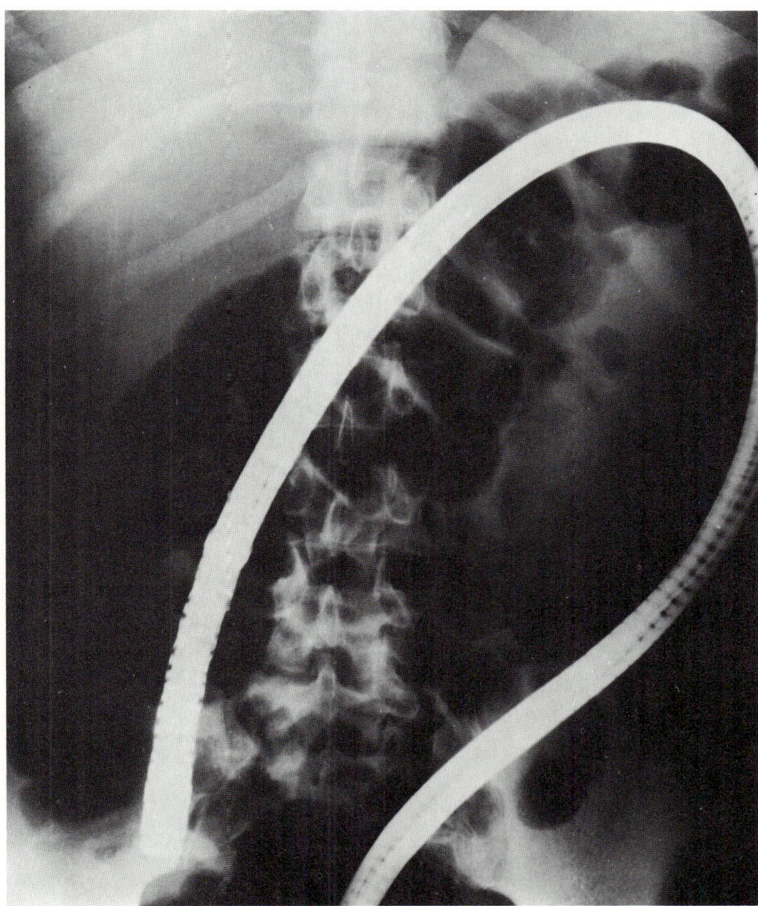

*Figure 7-11.   The cecum has been reached and the colon assumes an upside-down **U** shape.*

mesentery, and distention of loops. In any event, however long it may take to reach the cecum, that endpoint represents just the beginning of the diagnostic evaluation of the colon. It is on withdrawal of the colonoscope that the close observation of mucosal change is initiated. The time it takes for withdrawal of the instrument depends a good deal on the pathologic findings and the need for one or more polypectomies or mucosal biopsies. Withdrawal must be done slowly with appropriate maneuvers to be sure that all the wall of the bowel is examined. This may be difficult to do in the cecum, for example, because the tip of the colonoscope is so close to the medial wall of the colon, but by repositioning the patient a complete view may be obtained. On withdrawal from the flexures, seeing either side of the lesser curvature can be a problem. Indeed, the instrument may fall out of the flexure so fast that a good look is difficult. One must recognize that mucosal change or polypoid lesions can be overlooked in the flexure areas. Generally, the transverse colon and descending colon can be examined thoroughly, but on occasion a small polyp may be missed behind a haustral fold.

It is not an unusual experience to note the presence of a polyp in the colon on insertion of the colonoscope but to suffer considerable frustration in locating this polyp on withdrawal. This failure is due in part to the expectation that a polyp will be found at the same linear depth on withdrawal at which it was noted on insertion. On completion of total colonoscopy, the linear depth of the instrument is usually 80 or 90 cm once the colon has been straightened and pleated over the colonoscope. On withdrawal of the colonoscope even more shortening of the bowel occurs, and one may be surprised at finding a polyp in the distal descending colon at perhaps half the original linear extent at which it was noted on the way in.

Withdrawal should proceed with a circular motion of the tip to view the entire circumference of the bowel. When this does not bring the area completely into view, torsion of the instrument will achieve the panorama. In addition, it may be necessary to change the position of the patient from the left decubitus to the supine or prone position. Because of the prominence of the valves of the rectum, it may be particularly troublesome to examine both sides of these valves. If there is any question about the adequacy of the fiberoptic study, then the rectum should be reexamined with a rigid sigmoidoscope (although sigmoidoscopy should have been done previously as part of the routine diagnostic workup).

Cleaning the Colonoscope
Once the instrument is out of the colon, it should be washed with soap and water immediately. A gauze pad moistened in 70 percent alcohol is used to clean the head of the instrument, including the controls. The shaft may then be wiped down with an alcohol sponge and the tip of the instrument carefully wiped off. The suction channel is cleaned by aspirating a solution of glutaraldehyde through it. The biopsy channels are rinsed from the proximal end with the disinfecting solution, and then the biopsy-suction channels cleared by aspirating tap water through the system. The air-insufflation channel should be rinsed, and then dried by depressing the air insufflation button and expelling all the water. The colonoscope shaft is allowed to soak in glutaraldehyde for 10 minutes, after which it is rinsed and dried. Then the colonoscope should be hung in a tall cabinet specially adapted to receive the head of the colonoscope so that it hangs its full length to allow drainage of any fluid remaining in either channel.

Before the instrument is put away, however, it should be checked out to be sure that no mechanical problem has developed. The colonoscope should be evaluated for broken fibers and the presence of water that may have leaked into the lens compartment. The controls should be checked, and a determination of the responsiveness of the tip to flexing the up, down, right, and left control. Repairs to colonoscopic instruments are costly yet inevitable with frequent use. Starting a procedure with a malfunctioning colonoscope should be avoided by a system check immediately after cleaning by the assistant, and again before the next colonoscopy by the physician.

COLONOSCOPY FINDINGS
Benign Polyps
Because some polyps have malignant potential, it is important to distinguish the histologic types of polyps. The only way to accomplish this is to excise the polyp and study it microscopically. Colonoscopy permits pathologic study of virtually every polyp encountered, since polypectomy can be done for every polyp, except perhaps the large sessile tumors that can at least be biopsied. The different types of colon polyps are listed below.

1. Hyperplastic
2. Adenomatous
   a. Tubular
   b. Tubulovillous
   c. Villous
3. Hamartomatous
   a. Juvenile
   b. Peutz-Jegher
4. Inflammatory

The majority of polyps found in the colon are hyperplastic, and are characterized histologically by elongated, dilated crypts. The hyperplastic polyps occur most frequently in the rectum, measure less than 0.5 cm in diameter and have no malignant potential.

Adenomas, on the other hand, are a neoplastic type of polyp and are designated as tubular, tubulovillous, or villous, depending on the predominant histologic finding. The endoscopic appearance, for the most part, does not allow one to identify the nature of the adenoma, although the larger the polyp, the more likely it is that it will be villous. The surface appearance or the presence of a pedicle does not allow classification, but a small pedunculate polyp with a smooth surface is usually a tubular adenoma, whereas a large shaggy-surfaced sessile polyp is a villous adenoma (see Plate 44).

The adenomatous polyp has, according to Morson, definite malignant potential that increases with the size of the polyp and the degree of villous architecture. Thus, a villous adenoma over 2 cm in diameter has a 50 percent likelihood of having malignant change, contrasted to a one percent chance of cancer in a tubular adenoma less than 1 cm in size. The colonoscopist trained to remove polyps greater than 1 cm has the first real opportunity to reduce the death rate from colon cancer in the last 20 years.

Hamartomas occur in the Peutz-Jeghers syndrome, which consists of skin pigmentation and polyps of the gastrointestinal tract. Although most polyps are in the small intestine, they will occasionally be found in the colon; rarely are they restricted to the colon.

Juvenile polyps are also hamartomas found in patients under the age of twenty. Seventy-five percent of these polyps occur in the rectum and are found as a result of painless bleeding after defecation. The juvenile polyp is rarely larger than 2 cm, and has a smooth surface and spheric configuration (see Plates 45 and 46). Microscopically, there is cystic dilation of the glands that are separated one from the other by an abundance of lamina propria.

Other rare polypoid neoplasms such as lipoma (see Plate 47) or fibroma may also be found in the colon.

Inflammatory polyps include both ulcerative and granulomatous (Crohn's) colitis. The polyps may be solitary or diffuse and occur most often above the rectosigmoid junction. Polyps vary in size but are wormlike in appearance rather than pedunculate, and soft to forceps palpation (see Plate 48). The histology shows a picture of a variable inflammatory infiltrate distorting the mucosal architecture. The inflammatory polyp has no malignant potential but may be confused on barium enema study with an adenoma or cancer. Diffuse inflammatory polyps may, contrarily, mask the presence of an adenoma or cancer. Colonoscopic biopsy is needed at times to determine the nature of any suspicious polyp found in the setting of inflammatory bowel disease.

Malignant Polyps

Malignant polyps can be characterized as having in situ carcinoma (see Plate 49), which involves only the epithelial surface of the polyp, superficial carcinoma, which extends into the glandular structure of the polyp, or invasive carcinoma, which spreads into the pedicle and reaches the lymphatics.

Generally it is not possible to identify malignant changes endoscopically. Biopsy of a polyp is frowned on unless for some reason it is not possible to remove the polyp in toto. Polypectomy should always include the pedicle so that evaluation for invasive cancer can be made.

In familial polyposis of the colon, hundreds of adenomas appear in the second to third decade of life, to be followed in the third or fourth decade by the development of colon cancer, usually at more than one site. The adenomas are, for the most part, flat and small; they have, nevertheless, a high malignant potential.

Colon Cancer

From an endoscopic point of view, adenocarcinoma of the colon occurs as an ulcerating (see Plate 50), polypoid, or scirrhous lesion. The polypoid cancers are seen primarily in the ascending colon, while the ulcerating and scirrhous type are more frequently encountered in the left colon. Ordinarily, the diagnosis of colon cancer when established by barium enema does not require confirmation by colonoscopy. However, colonoscopy may be valuable to remove polyps that may not be included in the segment to be resected or to exclude a synchronous carcinoma.

Occasionally hemoccult positive stools may not be explained by sigmoidoscopy or barium enema and colonoscopy will identify a frank cancer of the colon. A surprisingly large fungating cancer in the cecum or a flat scirrhous tumor anywhere in the colon may be overlooked radiologically.

Inflammatory Bowel Disease

The colonoscopic differentiation of granulomatous and ulcerative colitis is not difficult in 75 percent of the patients, but 10 to 20 percent of the cases may not have the telltale signs to distinguish the specific inflammatory bowel disease.

Granulomatous (Crohn's) colitis is almost a certainty endoscopically when the rectum is spared and aphthoid linear ulcers are scattered through otherwise normal mucosa (see Plate 51). The mucosa may take on a nodular or cobblestone appearance at intervals throughout the colon. The mucosa is minimally friable and bleeding is not evident. The ileum may show ulcers and nodularity with Crohn's disease but no more than a diffuse erythema (so-called backwash ileitis) is seen with ulcerative colitis.

Ulcerative colitis is readily diagnosed when there is diffuse erythema, edema, and superficial ulceration of the rectum extending into the sigmoid and descending colon in a continuous fashion (see Plate 52). The mucosa is friable and there is usually fresh blood present in the lumen of the bowel as well as a purulent type of exudate. Ulcerative colitis may progress to involve the whole colon, but it does not extend into the ileum.

In a chronic phase of inflammatory bowel disease where the colon is tubular, the mucosa is nodular and there are numerous inflammatory polyps, the differentiation of ulcerative colitis from granulomatous colitis becomes quite difficult. Biopsy of the mucosa showing crypt abscess is more consistent with ulcerative colitis, and the finding of granulomas more consistent with granulomatous colitis, but neither histologic finding is specific for one or the other type of inflammatory bowel disease.

Other Colonic Diseases

Inflammatory bowel disease, of course, may be mimicked by other types of colitis. In particular, amebic colitis, when severe, may show changes quite similar to ulcerative colitis. However, the classic appearance for amebiasis of the rectum and sigmoid is that of discrete ulcers separated by normal-appearing mucosa. Of course, this diagnosis should be made by demonstration of the motile trophozooites in the exudate or by evidence of trophozooites in mucosal biopsies. The cecum is frequently involved by amebic infestation and ulcerations may be evident there as well as in the rectosigmoid area.

One should always consider the possibility of bacillary dysentery when the endoscopic picture in the distal colon appears to be that of ulcerative colitis. Stool cultures will provide a specific diagnosis.

Tuberculosis of the colon is rare in the United States. It affects primarily the ileocecal area where the thickening and edema of the submucosa result in superficial ulceration. Colonoscopic study will show a picture indistinguishable from Crohn's disease in the colon, but of course the microscopic presence of caseation necrosis within granulomas is characteristic of tuberculosis.

Radiation injury to the colon is becoming a more frequent problem as radiotherapy for pelvic cancer becomes more commonly part of cancer therapy. The endoscopic appearance is quite variable; colonoscopic biopsy may be of some help in the differentiation of colitis, but often the histologic findings are not specific.

POLYPECTOMY

Introduction

There is no question that pioneer work of Shinya and Wolff in the development of colonoscopic polypectomy has brought about a revolution in the management of colonic polyps. The numerous papers since 1969 cataloging the technique, indications, results, and complications have led to an adoption of this method across the country and the world. It is clear that the ease with which endoscopic polypectomy can be done is based on adequate training in diagnostic colonoscopy followed by close supervision of polypectomy technique. Shinya and Wolff claim and have the results to prove that proper attention to the details of polypectomy practice will virtually eliminate major complications. Nevertheless, a complication from polypectomy can happen, and the most experienced endoscopist must be prepared to handle the problem.

Indications, Contraindications, and Complications
The finding of a polyp with a diameter of 1 cm or larger on the barium enema study is an indication for colonoscopic polypectomy. Ordinarily, polyps smaller than that size can be handled by biopsy alone, particularly if sessile. However, some of the borderline-size polyps may be more conveniently removed with the polypectomy snare. The contraindications to the procedure are the same as outlined for diagnostic colonoscopy with the added proviso that a poor risk patient becomes even a worse candidate for surgical correction of postpolypectomy hemorrhage. A polyp that appears malignant and probably invasive should not be removed by colonoscopic polypectomy. A pedunculate polyp with a head diameter greater than 3 cm should only be removed by skilled and experienced endoscopists. A large, sessile polyp that will require removal in multiple pieces should not be handled by the neophyte colonoscopist.

The most common complication after polypectomy is bleeding. In the American Society for Gastrointestinal Endoscopy study, hemorrhage occurred in 68 patients from a total number of 5846 polypectomies. Ten perforations were also reported in this group of polypectomy patients. In the diagnostic cases representing three times as many cases, there were only five instances of hemorrhage and 35 of perforation. The complications of hemorrhage or perforation are basically related to inexperience of the examiner and inadequate visualization during polypectomy. One must be sure that the snare is not close to the base, does not include a piece of mucosa from the adjacent wall, and is completely snug about the whole circumference of the stalk. One must always be confident that the equipment is in top-notch condition in order to stay out of trouble. Electrocautery devices should be replaced after 10 or 12 polypectomies. If the wire breaks during polypectomy, it is almost always a signal for complication.

Instrumentation
The authors use the long bundle fiberoptic colonoscope for excision of colonic polyps primarily because a total colonoscopic procedure should, if possible, precede polypectomy. This avoids doing a double procedure on the patient. If an unexpected polyp should be found on a diagnostic study, however, and the patient has not been properly informed or prepared for polypectomy, a subsequent procedure may be done with the shorter scope. Long scopes with two channels that allow suction to be carried out at the time of polypectomy (or permit a bi-

opsy forceps to be passed along with the snare if there is some problem in looping the polyp) have an advantage, but are more difficult to use.

There are numerous snare and cautery devices available, all of which are based on the original design of Shinya and Wolff. The snare consists of single strand or braided wire of 0.5 mm in diameter, doubled over and inserted through a Teflon catheter of 2.7 mm outside diameter. The wire loop itself may measure anywhere from 2 to 5 cm in diameter (Fig. 2-20).

The electrocoagulating units are made by several companies, including ACMI, Olympus, Valley Laboratories, and Cameron-Miller Instrument Co. The electrosurgical unit works best when used with the manufacturer's snare. The authors have used (in the past) the Cameron-Miller unit (Model #807910), which provides a blended cutting and coagulating current, and will only operate if the circuit between the unit, snare, and grounded patient is intact. The SurgiStat model of Valley Laboratories is being used more often because of its excellent engineering and safety control (see Fig. 7-12). A patient with a cardiac pacemaker cannot have polypectomy because of the risk of pacemaker malfunction.

Preparation

The patient is prepared in the fashion previously described for diagnostic colonoscopy. For polypectomy, however, an additional day on a liquid diet is advisable to insure a clean colon. Should there be fecal residual in the colon, the procedure should not be done; it should be deferred until proper preparation has been accomplished. When one has gained experience and confidence in his technique, then polypectomy for small polyps on a stalk can be performed on the outpatient basis. For large polyps on short pedicles, or where multiple polyps will be re-

Figure 7-12. The Valley Lab electrosurgical unit.

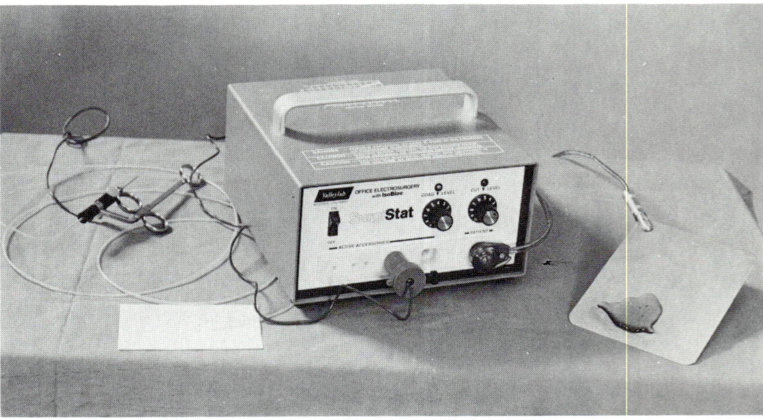

moved, or in patients who are an increased risk, the polypectomy is best performed on hospitalized patients. Appropriate studies should be done prior to polypectomy; these include blood count, coagulation screening, blood typing, crossmatch, and appropriate blood chemistry studies. These studies are, of course, in addition to the usual baseline determinations made in any hospitalized patient; namely, a complete history and physical examination with chest x-ray and electrocardiogram. The patient should be fully informed of the nature of the procedure of the polypectomy and be aware of the risks involved.

Technique

The colonoscopy is usually done without the benefit of fluoroscopy unless there is anticipation of difficulty traversing the sigmoid loops because of previous surgery or inflammatory reaction, or because of the necessity of being sure that the cecum has been entered. The patient assumes the left lateral recumbent position and the instrument is advanced as it would be for a diagnostic study to the cecum. If difficulty is encountered in advancing beyond the site of the polyp, however, the diagnostic procedure is discontinued so as not to jeopardize the possibility of removing the polyp. Under those circumstances, a total colonoscopy will be done at a later date to exclude other polyps.

Although the diagnostic study can be done without assistance, for polypectomy an experienced assistant should be present. The endoscopist should have a strategy based on the barium enema findings prior to polypectomy. If there is more than one polyp to be removed, the wisest approach is to remove the proximal one, first bringing that polyp out by applying suction to it with the tip of the instrument and then returning for the distal polyp. If there is a large polyp (of 3 cm or more in diameter), however, this should be taken first and the other small polyps removed at a subsequent examination. Polyps larger than 3 cm carry increased risks from colonoscopic polypectomy, and only those with considerable experience should attempt to remove them.

When the polyp is in view, a rapid appraisal of its shape, size, and length of its stalk should be made. At this point the decision must be made as to whether the polyp can be removed in one piece by transecting the stalk, or whether it will have to be taken off in multiple pieces. The polyp may be manipulated by the tip of the catheter and suction insufflation may be applied so as to change the direction of the polyp in the lumen. In addition, the patient's position may be altered to provide better access to the polyp. Most polyps are pedunculate, and the usual approach is to loop the wire over the polyp and tighten it about the stalk at approximately 1 cm from the mucosal surface of the bowel wall. The wire should not be tightened until the level of transection has been precisely determined. Prior to application of the coagulating current, the electrocoagulation unit should have been turned on with a setting appropriate for the unit being used. In addition, of course, the patient will have been previously grounded by an armband or ground plate depending on the unit used. A systematic check of the electrocoagulation circuit should be done before attaching the wire from the unit to the handle of the electrocoagulation snare. It goes without saying of course that basic principles of electrosurgery should be understood by the endoscopist prior to participating in any polypectomy procedure.

A clear view of the polyp is essential. This requires adequate insufflation of the bowel and manipulation of the stalk to bring the head of the polyp away from the wall if possible. The question of using carbon dioxide for insufflation during polypectomy has been raised because of the danger of explosion of combustible gases in the bowel. This risk has been probably overemphasized. There are now several studies that show that with adequate bowel preparation and repeated aspiration and insufflation of the bowel with air, any detectable concentration of combustible gases is well below the explosive level, but carbon dioxide insufflation does add an unquestionable measure of safety.

Now back to the polyp where the snare wire has been put around the stalk approximately 1 cm from the wall of the bowel. If the stalk is not long enough, the wire loop should be placed around the midportion of the pedicle. The snare wire is then applied snugly but not tightly, and the coagulation current put on for a few seconds. During the time of application of the current, if the polyp is not free in the lumen of the bowel but rests against the bowel wall at one point or another, an oscillating movement should be applied to the catheter so that no current is conducted to a point of contact. From the aspect of transmission of the coagulating current to the bowel wall, it is better to have a large surface of the polyp resting on the bowel wall than a single point touching the bowel wall. It is usually possible to identify a narrow band of coagulation on either side of the wire and, on seeing that, another short burst of coagulation current will permit the endoscopist to close the loop and transect the stalk of the polyp. It is not necessary and probably unwise to tighten the snare about the stalk to strangle the polyp before snare electrocoagulation. Small polyps can be inadvertently pulled off the wall in that fashion, or the thicker stalks may be cut into and bleed, obscuring and interfering with a subsequent coagulation.

Following closure of the snare, the polyp will fall into the lumen and the coagulated stalk is visible. There may be some blood that has oozed from the polyp itself. Should there be bleeding from the stalk, the character of hemorrhage should be noted. If it is a moderate ooze it is best to leave well enough alone, since this type of bleeding will sub-side spontaneously. If there is an active pumping of blood from the stalk, however, then it is reasonable to take the loop and encircle the stalk, tightening it so that the bleeding is stopped, and then applying a coagulation current again. If the remaining stalk is not long enough for this, a coagulating probe may be used to control bleeding from a short stub of a stalk. It is not wise to attempt coagulation if there is not an adequate pedicle projecting from the bowel wall since nothing will be accomplished if perforation compounds the bleeding complication. Although the tip of the snare may be used for coagulation hemostasis, it is best not to use this but to use the specially designed coagulation probe.

When sufficient observation of the coagulated stalk indicates that there is no bleeding, then with the catheter removed from the biopsy channel, the colonoscope tip is applied to the polyp and, with suction, the polyp is brought out with the colonoscope. If the polyp is small and soft, use less suction and change the suction bottle so that if the small polyp is aspirated into the channel it can be easily collected. With large polyps there will be a red-out as the polyp occludes the tip of the colonoscope. If the red-out does not persist as the polyp is being brought out, then it means that the polyp has undoubtedly fallen off and must be relocated. A large polyp often drops off repeatedly, particularly when being brought around the flexures; these polyps can be retrieved later on with a tap water enema. Another technique is to administer 500 ml of tap water through a catheter placed into the biopsy channel in the segment of the bowel where the polyp fell off. The patient will pass the polyp with the enema fluid soon after the completion of the study. It may not be possible to pull large polyps through the anus with the colonoscope, but if the patient bears down at that time they will be expelled. Sometimes, the polyp must be removed from the rectum after the procedure by passing a rigid sigmoidoscope and grasping it with forceps.

Some endoscopists have been reinserting the colonoscope to view the site of polypectomy again. This appears to be an unnecessary maneuver if the coagulated stalk has been adequately viewed and a determination has been made that there is no bleeding, or at least no bleeding that requires additional therapeutic effort. In patients in whom the original intubation has been difficult and particularly when the procedure has gone on for some time, to recolonoscope merely to inspect the stalk is inconsiderate to the patient and a waste of time. If there is a second polyp to be retrieved, however, then it is not unreasonable to examine the site of polypectomy of the first polyp if it is in proximity.

A second intubation for polypectomy is generally easier than the first because the bowel has already been straightened out. However, the patient may be restless by this time, not only because of the duration of the procedure but because the sedation is no longer effective. Therefore, one should remember to give additional medication during the procedure via the intravenous fluid running into the right arm. Also at this point, even if there is considerably more peristaltic activity of the colon, the temptation to give anticholinergic medication should be resisted. These drugs tend to create a hypotonic bowel which becomes overdistended with air. If severe spasm is encountered, intravenous glucagon 0.5 to 1.0 mg may be given, and this appears to be effective for its duration of action, which is much shorter than anticholinergic agents.

When multiple polyps are to be removed, then the location of each polyp should be carefully recorded and each polyp should be submitted as a separate specimen. How many polyps should be removed at one session depends a good deal on the tolerance of the patient, the type of polyps to be removed, and the ease of the procedure. The authors have removed as many as five polyps in a single session, but this may mean reintubating the patient for each polyp. Even though the patient may not seem to mind, it may be quite a tour de force for the endoscopist.

When the polyp is delivered, it can be photographed with a Polaroid camera so that a permanent record is attached to the patient's history. The polyp is fixed in formalin solution and examined by serial section to determine the presence of epithelial atypia or frank cancer which may be within the polyp or invading the stalk. The histology of the polyp cannot be determined by looking at the gross specimen, and at this stage it is fair to advise the patient that it is probably benign, but a final determination must be made by the pathologist.

Postpolypectomy Procedure
Following polypectomy the inpatient is kept at bedrest for several hours with vital signs being checked. If there is a suggestion of bleeding, then the intravenous fluid is maintained throughout the night. A patient is explicitly requested to examine all stools and report bleeding. If bleeding is observed, an expectant approach is best since very few patients require surgical intervention. If no bleeding has occurred over the next 12 to 24 hours, then the clear liquid diet is discontinued and the patient is discharged to convalesce for another two days. The patient would be wise to avoid strenuous exertion or heavy lifting for an additional week. To have the patient return in a few weeks for progress colonoscopy simply to look at the site of polypectomy is an unnecessary effort and expense. It is our policy, however, that a patient who has had a polyp removed should have a progress colonoscopy in a year; if at that time there is no evidence of polyp formation, then he

need not be reexamined for two to three years, at which time a double contrast barium enema could be done for survey purposes.

Undoubtedly colonoscopy represents a major advance in endoscopic practice. But more than its diagnostic role, the therapeutic application of removal of polyps has had a significant impact on the practice of surgery. For all practical purposes, laparotomy for removal of colon polyps is a matter of history. With a 7 percent incidence of malignancy in polyps, it is anticipated that the removal of polyps will have a salutory effect on the incidence of colon cancer and for the first time in the last 20 years, bring about a reduction of deaths due to colon cancer.

SELECTED READINGS

Appel, M.F.   Preoperative and postoperative colonoscopy for colorectal carcinoma. *Dis. Colon Rectum* 19:664, 1976.

Axon, A.T.R., et al.   Disinfection of gastrointestinal fibre endoscopes. *Lancet* 1:656, 1974.

Knutson, C.O., Schrock, L.C., and Polk, H.C.   Polypoid lesions of the proximal colon: Comparison of experiences with removal at laparotomy and by colonoscopy. *Ann. Surg.* 179:657, 1974.

Morson, B.C.   *The Pathogenesis of Colorectal Cancer.* Philadelphia: Saunders, 1978.

Norfleet, R.G., et al.   Does bacteremia follow colonoscopy? *Gastroenterology* 70:20, 1976.

Overholt, B.F.   Colonoscopy: A review. *Gastroenterology* 68:1308, 1975.

Ragins, H., Shinya, H., and Wolff, W.I.   The explosive potential of colonic gas during colonoscopic electrosurgical polypectomy. *Surg. Gynecol. Obstet.* 138:554, 1974.

Rogers, G.H.G., et al.   Complications of flexible fiberoptic colonoscopy and polypectomy. *Gastrointest. Endosc.* 22:73, 1975.

Schmitt, M.G., Jr., et al.   Diagnostic colonoscopy: An assessment of the clinical indications. *Gastroenterology* 69:765, 1975.

Suarez, A., et al.   Bacteremia associated with colonoscopy. *Henry Ford Hospital Medical Journal* 26:59, 1978.

Tawile, N.T., Priest, R.J., and Schuman, B.M.   Colonoscopy in inflammatory bowel disease. *Gastrointest. Endosc.* 22:1, 1975.

Waye, J.D.   Colitis, cancer and colonoscopy. *Med. Clin. North Am.* 61:1977.

Wolff, W.I., et al.   Comparison of colonoscopy and the contrast enema in 500 patients with colorectal disease. *Am. J. Surg.* 129:181, 1975.

Wolff, W.I., and Shinya, H.   Polypectomy via the fiberoptic colonoscope. *N. Engl. J. Med.* 288:329, 1973.

CHAPTER 8

THERAPEUTIC ENDOSCOPY

Gastrointestinal fiberscopes are used primarily as diagnostic tools, but therapeutic applications have become very important. Therapeutic procedures currently in use include

1. Foreign body removal
2. Polypectomy
3. Placement of tubes through strictures or surgical anastomoses
4. Dilation of stricture
5. Suture removal
6. Sphincterotomy and removal of gallstones
7. Control of gastrointestinal hemorrhage

FOREIGN BODY REMOVAL

Foreign bodies in the esophagus and stomach can be removed with a forward-viewing esophagogastroduodenoscope. A standard-sized instrument should be used so that adequate grasping forceps, polypectomy snares, dormier baskets, and "polyp graspers" can be passed through the biopsy channel of the instrument. In children, the most common foreign bodies are coins, buttons, toys, marbles, or safety pins; and most of the foreign bodies are impacted in the upper esophagus at the cricopharyngeal junction. In adults the foreign bodies are meat bolus, bones, dentures, nails, or needles; these generally become impacted at the site of the predisposing lesion or in the lower esophagus. Most foreign bodies will pass spontaneously, but pointed objects should be extracted, if possible, because of the possibility of perforation (see Fig. 8-1 and Plate 53). Large foreign bodies that do not pass the pylorus will also need to be removed. It is wise to remove the foreign body with the patient in a head-down position, so that if it should get free of the grasping tool as it passes the hypopharynx, it will not drop back by gravity into the trachea.

Keys or other objects that have holes in them can be removed by passing a short piece of cotton tape or silk through the hole with the forceps, and removing the object by grasping the tape with the biopsy forceps. If the hole is large enough to admit the biopsy forceps, then the object may be withdrawn by opening the biopsy forceps once it has passed through the hole. Needles can be grasped at the head and withdrawn into the biopsy channel. The needle is then brought out within the endoscope (Fig. 8-1 and Plate 53). Open safety pins should

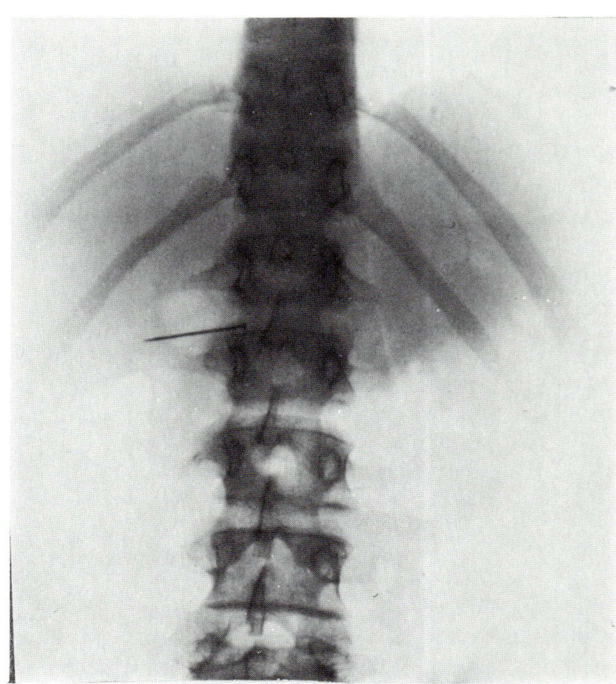

Figure 8-1. X-ray of abdomen of a 13-year-old girl showing a sewing needle in the duodenal bulb.

be removed by grasping the blunt end with a forceps and bringing the pin out with the point directed caudad.

Sharp objects such as razor blades must be withdrawn from the stomach within a plastic sleeve that covers the endoscope, sleeve and endoscope having been passed in together. Where several sharp objects are present, the plastic sleeve allows multiple passages of the endoscope for withdrawal. The sleeve protects the pharynx and esophagus and avoids the risk of aspiration of the foreign body.

Impaction of meat in the distal esophagus is a common occurrence; if one is sure that no obstructing lesion is distal to the meat impaction, the meat may be pushed into the stomach. Without that knowledge, however, meat must be removed by grasping it in toto with a snare or a four-pronged polyp grasper, or by breaking it up into small pieces with a large biopsy forceps. Bones in the esophagus or stomach should be crushed into smaller pieces if at all possible.

Particularly in the postoperative stomach, gastric bezoars composed of vegetable fibers or other concretions may cause symptoms. In the past it was necessary to operate in order to remove these bezoars, but successful treatment can now be provided by mechanical disruption and lavage with saline or papain. Direct injection of papain into the bezoar through a catheter is also a successful approach.

POLYPECTOMY

Snare excision of polyps using electrocoagulation can be performed in any place the fiberscope can reach. It has been most frequently performed in the colon, where the vast majority of polyps arise. The technique described in Chapter 7 applies as well to polypectomy in the stomach and duodenum.

PLACEMENT OF TUBES THROUGH STRICTURES OR SURGICAL ANASTOMOSES

Feeding catheters have been positioned through a surgical anastomosis or an esophageal stricture via the biopsy channel of a fiberoptic esophagogastroduodenoscope. When a tube is pulled down with the endoscope, it should have an inflatable balloon at the end so that it is not withdrawn during removal of the endoscope. To place a Miller-Abbott tube through a narrowed gastrojejunostomy, for example, it is possible to grasp with the biopsy forceps the end of the silk tied to the balloon of the Miller-Abbott tube. The endoscope and biopsy forceps are placed beyond the anastomosis or stricture and, after the desired location is reached, the balloon of the Miller-Abbott tube is inflated so that the tube is not pulled back as the endoscope is withdrawn.

Another technique reported by Morrissey utilized five rubber bands, tied at intervals of a few centimeters at the distal end of the tube to be put into position. The most distal rubber band is grasped by the forceps, and the tube is advanced to the desired position in the stomach or, more commonly, the duodenum. The endoscope is withdrawn somewhat, and the second rubber band is grasped with the forceps and advanced further into the hollow viscus. In this way the tube is slowly advanced as the endoscope is withdrawn, so that the tube remains in place and is not pulled out with the endoscope.

DILATION OF STRICTURES

Esophageal strictures can be dilated with a pediatric endoscope under direct vision at the time of esophagoscopy. This may be followed by progressive dilation with tapered mercury-filled bougies.

Tight strictures are handled by passing a fine wire through the biopsy channel of a fiberoptic esophagoscope, and guiding the obturator-tipped wire through the stricture. When the wire is coiled in the fundus of the stomach, the endoscope can be removed, leaving the wire in place. Eder-Puestow dilators of successively larger calibers are then passed over the guidewire.

A narrowed gastroenterostomy stoma can be dilated by passage of a pediatric endoscope followed by a standard endoscope. This should be done without excessive force, to avoid a rupture of the anastomosis.

SUTURE REMOVAL

Suture material protrusion at sites of anastomosis is not uncommon. For the most part these protrusions are asymptomatic, but occasionally sutures may result in ulceration with consequent bleeding or infection. If these sutures are associated with ulceration, they must be removed with a suture-cutting forceps if the ulcer is to heal. Other sutures may be easily pulled out with a biopsy forceps. Occasionally sutures fixed within the gastric wall do not yield to mechanical traction, and must be removed by electrocoagulating the visible segment of the suture, then pulling it out at one end.

PAPILLOTOMY AND REMOVAL OF GALLSTONES

After endoscopic retrograde cholangiopancreatography became commonplace, it was obvious that selective cannulation of the common bile duct made possible techniques to alleviate bile duct obstruction. As experience with ERCP increased, skilled endoscopists devised therapeutic maneuvers to remove stones from the biliary tree. First, it was evident that small stones and biliary sludge could be flushed from the bile duct merely by retrograde irrigation. Another technique involved introduction of a cannula with an inflatable balloon at the tip and, following distention of the balloon proximal to the stone, withdrawal of the stone with the balloon. Based on practice with ureteral stones, innovative endoscopists extracted small stones from the common duct by means of collapsible ureteral baskets introduced through the cannula.

The mere introduction of the cannula into the common bile duct allows flushing out of stones smaller than 4 mm with contrast medium. Stones larger than 4 mm can be grasped with a ureteral basket, but attempting to pull such a stone out through an intact papilla can lead to entrapment of the basket unless the stone can be crushed.

For the management of choledocholithiasis in postcholecystectomy patients, or in high-risk surgical candidates with intact gallbladder, an endoscopically performed incision of the papilla of Vater was developed, facilitating spontaneous passage of relatively large common bile duct stones. The technique of papillotomy, as initiated by Kawai and Sohma in Japan and Demling in Germany, allows guided incision of the papilla to a length of 0.5 to 1.0 cm with further extension into the duodenal wall as necessary for a total length of up to 3 cm. The longer incisions are more properly defined as sphincterotomy (see Fig. 8-2).

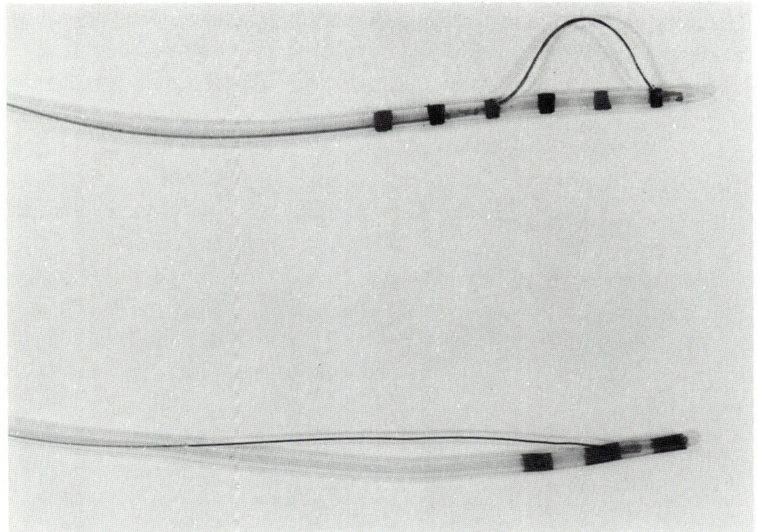

Figure 8-2.   Two types of papillotomes.

One method requires insertion of a catheter that contains a thin steel wire into the papilla. Traction is then placed on the wire, which is exposed from the tip of the catheter for a distance of 3 cm, to retroflex the tip so that the wire becomes taut. An electrocoagulation current is then passed through the wire, so that cutting and coagulation may be carried out under direct vision. The length of the incision varies with the size of the stone or stones to pass. Another method of incising the papilla involves advancing the papillotome into the papilla under direct vision. This is a more popular technique in Japan, but in other centers it is sometimes done as a "precut" to allow cannulation of the common bile duct and a traction papillotomy.

In addition to the management of common bile duct stones, other indications include cholangitis related to obstruction by stones or stenosis, and distal stricture of the common bile duct. Papillary stenosis is considered an indication by some endoscopists, although the very existence of the diagnosis remains controversial. Endoscopic papillotomy should not be done in the face of a coagulation disorder, a long stricture of the common duct, certain anatomic abnormalities, anomalies of the bile ducts, or acute pancreatitis.

The complications that might be encountered in endoscopic papillotomy include bleeding, pancreatitis, cholangitis, and perforation. The overall mortality reported in Europe and in the United States is between 1.0 and 1.5 percent. In view of the fact that many of the patients are elderly and have other serious illness, this compares favorably with the surgical mortality, which, in this type of patient, may be as high as 8 percent.

A compilation of several European series, documenting over 1500 endoscopic papillotomy and sphincterotomy cases, showed that 94 percent were successfully completed, with spontaneous passage of stones in 54 percent. Extraction was required in 32 percent. Fourteen percent of the cases were failures or incomplete procedures. In the total group there were 16 deaths, for a mortality rate of 1.1 percent.

It is evident that endoscopists who have had a large experience in ERCP can, on the basis of definitive diagnosis, proceed with a therapeutic procedure—be it flushing, extraction, papillotomy, or sphincterotomy with or without extraction—which will result in complete resolution of the problem of choledocholithiasis with a minimum hospital stay and an acceptable morbidity and mortality rate.

CONTROL OF GASTROINTESTINAL HEMORRHAGE

Modern technology makes direct endoscopic identification of bleeding upper gastrointestinal lesions possible in over 85 percent of cases. Experiments with animals employing laser beams and electrocoagulation have been conducted with subsequent clinical use of both endoscopically. These techniques applied to patients with massive hemorrhage unresponsive to conventional noninvasive therapy may save lives, especially in the aged, in patients with serious liver disease, and in severely septic patients. Whether these methods should be used in patients who are not poor surgical risks has yet to be determined.

The endoscopic modalities to control gastrointestinal hemorrhage are (1) electrocoagulation, (2) laser coagulation, (3) injection of sclerosing agents, (4) topical spray of hemostatic agents, and (5) application of hemoclips.

Electrocoagulation

CLINICAL EXPERIENCE.   Over a four and one-half year period, we have examined more than 800 patients with upper gastrointestinal bleeding. Thirty-one severely ill patients, with actively bleeding lesions in the stomach and esophagus, have undergone electrocoagulation. Based on data obtained in experimental animals, 40 watts were applied over one to three seconds in one to five applications. Electrocoagulation was successful in stopping the bleeding initially in 30 of the 31 patients (see Table 8-1). One patient with a gastric ulcer was bleeding very briskly, and electrocoagulation could not be achieved. A patient with acute erosive gastritis due to sepsis rebled 24 hours later, and a patient with chronic gastric ulcer and another with telangiectasia rebled 36 hours later.

Diagnosis	Number of Patients	Mean Units of Blood Transfused	Rebled
AGML	12	4.8	2
Mallory-Weiss syndrome	7	3.6	0
Marginal ulcer	5	5.7	0
Gastric ulcer	5	4.4	1
Gastric polyps	1	2.0	0
Esophageal ulcer	1	9.0	0

Table 8-1.   Clinical Experience with Electrocoagulation

CASE STUDY.   A 45-year-old man developed massive hematemesis after severe coughing. He had had a splenorenal shunt for bleeding esophageal varices one and a half years ago. He required nine units of blood over a ten-hour period. He was bleeding so rapidly that endoscopy could not be done initially; under general anesthesia, following vigorous irrigation of the stomach and esophagus, endoscopy revealed an esophageal tear with a pumping vessel. No esophageal varices were found. Electrocoagulation with a monopolar electrode produced immediate hemostasis He recovered completely with no recurrent bleeding. A white-based esophageal ulcer was seen one week after electrocoagulation by endoscopic examination.

Hemostasis by means of electrocoagulation has proven to be a safe and reliable method in the animal model, and may be extended to carefully selected patients. Neither perforation nor excessive necrosis of the gastric or esophageal mucosa will occur if precautions are taken to avoid excessive coagulation. Current requirements for coagulation vary with the condition of the mucosal area to be treated. The principles underlying electrocoagulation, as excellently outlined by Curtiss, must be understood before embarking on this mode of therapy.

Laser Coagulation

Laser is very intense light that, when absorbed by tissue, generates heat and thus coagulates blood and tissue proteins. Argon laser therapy is limited in severe bleeding because the light is absorbed by the surrounding red blood rather than by the underlying open artery. A technique was devised whereby a jet of carbon dioxide gas coaxial to the laser beam blew away the overlying blood and allowed the laser energy to be deposited on the bleeding vessel. This technique has been successfully applied in patients by Fruhmorgen and Waitman.

The Nd-Yag laser radiation is transmitted through a quartz fiber. Unlike the argon laser, Nd-Yag laser radiation is not absorbed by blood since it emits in the invisible near-infrared range rather than in the green spectral range. On the other hand, the penetration depth of radiation into the dog's stomach wall is five times greater with the Nd-Yag (0.36 mm argon as opposed to 1.7 mm Nd-Yag). In spite of this greater depth of penetration, Kiefhaber's clinical experience has not shown any greater incidence of perforation than has occurred with argon laser therapy.

Injection of Sclerosing Agents
Transendoscopic needles are available to inject solutions into perivenal mucosa or into the veins themselves. Sclerosing agents, such as 5 percent morrhuate sodium and ethylolamine oleate (Varistab), have been used to treat esophageal varices. Extensive experimental work by one of the authors [C.S.] showed the effectiveness of 5 percent sodium morrhuate in thrombosing the bleeding varix.

Hemoclips
Hemoclips have been applied via the endoscope to a bleeding vessel. Hayashi in Japan attempted hemoclip application in 24 bleeding peptic ulcer patients with 11 successes. It requires great skill to position the clip, and it is unlikely that this technique will become popular in view of the operative difficulties and limited applicability.

SELECTED READINGS

Classen, M., and Roesch, W.   Endoscopic cutting of persisting suture material. *Gastrointest. Endosc.* 20:130, 1974.

Classen, M., et al.   Operative and therapeutic techniques. In K.F.R. Shiller, (ed.), *Clin. Gastroenterol.* 553:7, 1978.

Curtiss, L.E.   High frequency currents in endoscopy: A review of principles and precautions. *Gastrointest. Endosc.* 20:9, 1973.

Dwyer, R.M., et al.   Gastric hemostasis by laser phototherapy in man. *J.A.M.A.* 236:1383, 1976.

Fruhmorgen, P., et al.   The first successful endoscopic laser coagulations of bleeding and potential bleeding lesions in the human gastrointestinal tract. *Gastrointest. Endosc.* 22:225, 1976.

Gaisford, W.D.   A new prototype 2-channel upper gastrointestinal operating fiberscope. *Gastrointest. Endosc.* 22:148, 1976.

Gold, M.H., Patterson, T.E., and Green, G.I.   Cellulase bezoar injection: A new endoscopic technique. *Gastrointest. Endosc.* 22:220, 1976.

Katon, R.M.   Experimental control of gastrointestinal hemorrhage via the endoscope: A new era dawns. *Gastroenterology* 70:272, 1976.

Kiefhaber, P., Nath, G., and Moritz, K.   Endoscopical control of massive gastrointestinal hemorrhage by irradiation with a high-power neodymium YAG laser. *Prog. Surg.* 15:140, 1977.

Koch, H.   Operative endoscopy. *Gastrointest. Endosc.* 24:65, 1977.

Koch, H., et al.   Endoscopic papillotomy. *Gastroenterology* 73:1393, 1977.

Olsen, H., Lawrence, W., and Bernstein, R.   Fiberendoscopic removal of foreign bodies from the upper gastrointestinal tract. A simple and consistent method using a snare. *Gastrointest. Endosc.* 21:58, 1974.

Papp, J.P., Fox, S.M. and Nalbandean, R.M.   Endoscopic electrocoagulation of upper gastrointestinal hemorrhage. *J.A.M.A.* 236:2076, 1976.

Safrany, L. Duodenoscopic sphincterotomy and gallstone removal. *Gastroenterology* 72:338, 1977.

Silverstein, V.E., et al.   Endoscopic laser treatment III: The development and testing of a gas-jet-assisted argon laser waveguide in control of bleeding experimental ulcers. *Gastroenterology* 74:232, 1978.

Sugawa, C., et al.   Electrocoagulation of bleeding in the upper part of the gastrointestinal tract. A preliminary experimental clinical report. *Arch. Surg.* 110:975, 1975.

Zimmon, D.A.   Endoscopic management of biliary calculi. *Hosp. Pract.* 13:103–114, 1978.

CHAPTER 9

FIBEROPTIC ENDOSCOPY IN INFANTS AND CHILDREN

Although fiberoptic endoscopy has become well established in adult patients, its use in infants and children is not common. Obviously there is less frequent indication for the procedure, since children have a smaller incidence of gastrointestinal disease that cannot be explained by the usual radiologic studies. In small hospitals where only a standard endoscope is available, endoscopy has been deferred when it might have provided important diagnostic information. The investment in a pediatric instrument, however, for the relatively few cases where endoscopy is indicated is not reasonable for the average institution; referral centers should be available to handle those cases.

UPPER GASTROINTESTINAL ENDOSCOPY

There is a select group of pediatric patients for whom upper gastrointestinal endoscopy is definitely indicated. In the management of upper gastrointestinal bleeding, a need for an early diagnosis is just as important in children as it is in adults. Children with recurrent or persistent abdominal pain unexplained by a barium study of the upper gastrointestinal tract will benefit from upper GI endoscopy, even if only to confirm a negative barium study. A potentially penetrating foreign body in the esophagus, stomach, or duodenum, or any foreign body that has been in the stomach for a few weeks should be removed endoscopically if at all possible. An inconclusive upper GI series may require gastroscopy for definition of the problem. The early detection of esophageal varices in childhood chronic hepatitis or cirrhosis is important in management, and can best be made by esophagoscopy. Finally, the management of esophageal strictures due to chemical burns requires esophagoscopy during both the acute and chronic phases of disease.

Instrumentation

Although the adult flexible fiberbronchoscope was first used for neonates and small infants for examination of the upper gastrointestinal tract, it did not prove entirely satisfactory. In recent years, the pediatric instruments of several manufacturers have been well tolerated by children over the age of two. These instruments measure 9 mm in diameter, and have a four-way angled tip that allows a complete examination of the esophagus, stomach, and duodenum. Any child over the age of 10 will tolerate the standard upper gastrointestinal endoscope readily.

Premedication and Anesthesia

As experience is gained in endoscopy of children, the need for general anesthesia declines. Most children over 12 years of age will do well with a combination of diazepam and meperidine in appropriate dosage for their weight. Moreover, there are a substantial number of children between 6 and 12 who will be able to accept endoscopy with premedication alone. These children should be done in an operating room suite, however, where endotracheal intubation and general anesthesia can be carried out if required. When foreign bodies are to be removed, it is wise to use general anesthesia so that maximum cooperation is achieved; with endotracheal intubation there is no risk of aspiration of the retrieved foreign body.

Procedure and Technique

If the patient is under general anesthesia, the endoscope can be passed with the child in the supine position, or the child can be moved into the left lateral position as usual. It is best to pass the gastroscope under direct vision behind the endotracheal tube into the esophagus. Once this maneuver is completed the remainder of the examination is carried out in the usual way. One must be careful not to overinflate the stomach, since the patient will not voluntarily belch air. Nor will there be any indication of discomfort from undue insufflation. The pediatric instrument is quite flexible, and at times there will be difficulty when it curls up in the fundus, but this provides an opportunity to inspect the fundus and cardiac area of the stomach before proceeding to examine the body, pylorus, and duodenum. The stomach should be deflated before the instrument is removed.

In a study by Liebman of 53 patients aged two months to 18 years, 20 required general anesthesia. Six of 27 patients with unexplained abdominal pain had gastric or duodenal ulcers, and 17 of 18 patients with upper gastrointestinal bleeding had an identifiable lesion.

In another study by Ament and Christie, six foreign bodies were removed under general anesthesia with the flexible panendoscope without complication.

COLONOSCOPY

Instruments

Most children will tolerate the single-channel medium colonoscope. In infants a pediatric endoscope can be used, although it will require thorough mechanical cleansing and gas sterilization for subsequent oral use. Our experience in children has been primarily with the Olympus CF-MB instrument, which has proved to be quite satisfactory for children over two years of age.

Indications

The most frequent indication for colonoscopy is the presence of gross blood in the stool, and failure to make a specific diagnosis by means of sigmoidoscopy or barium enema. Of course if a polyp has been identified by barium enema, colonoscopic polypectomy might be indicated. Colonoscopy for the explanation of prolonged lower abdominal pain appears to be of as little value in children as it is in adults. On occasion it may be important to do colonoscopy in order to determine the linear extent and intensity of inflammatory bowel disease. In teenagers who are related to patients with familial polyposis, colonoscopy might be used to establish the presence of multiple small polyps if the barium enema study is not conclusive.

Preparation

Ordinarily children require little in the way of laxation for a good colon preparation. A clear liquid diet 24 to 48 hours before the procedure, one ounce of Milk of Magnesia once or twice the day before, and a small tap water enema the morning of colonoscopy are usually sufficient. Most children tolerate colonoscopy remarkably well, requiring only premedication with diazepam or meperidine. General anesthesia may be required in preteenagers for polypectomy in order to obtain maximum cooperation. Obviously, endotracheal intubation is not necessary for colonoscopic examination.

Technique

The procedure is done in the usual lateral decubitus position. Ordinarily there is no difficulty in advancing the instrument under direct visualization, since the bowel loops are quite mobile and previous pelvic inflammatory disease or abdominal surgery is highly unlikely. Excessive insufflation of air is avoided by suctioning out the colon at regular intervals, and observing the abdomen carefully for undue distention.

It may be helpful to do colonoscopy under fluoroscopy in infants, since they tend to have a redundant sigmoid colon that may be difficult to straighten and shorten with the usual techniques. The excessive mobility of the colon may place undue stress on the wall. Serosal tears have been noted in children who have had laparotomy after colonoscopy. Moreover, the colonic wall of infants is thin and subject to perforation unless the most careful and gentle intubation is carried out.

Polypectomy

Most polypoid lesions of the colon in children are juvenile polyps. It is probably not necessary to remove these polyps if they are asymptomatic, since the majority of them eventually slough off. In children who are bleeding from polyps, however, colonoscopic polypectomy is definitely indicated for the small percentage that occurs beyond the rectosigmoid area (see Plate 54). The technique of colonoscopic polypectomy in children does not differ from that employed for adults.

SELECTED READINGS

Akasaka, Y., et al.   Endoscopy in pediatric patients with upper gastrointestinal bleeding. *Gastrointest. Endosc.* 23:199, 1977.

Ament, M.E., and Christie, D.L.   Upper gastrointestinal fiberoptic endoscopy in pediatric patients. *Gastroenterology* 72:1244, 1977.

Dyepes, M.T., Smith, L.E., and Ament, M.E.   Fiberoptic endoscopy and upper gastrointestinal series: Comparative analysis in infants and children. *Am. J. Roentgenol.* 128:53, 1977.

Gans, S.L., et al.   Pediatric endoscopy with flexible fiberscopes. *J. Pediatr. Surg.* 10(3):375, 1975.

Holgersen, L.O., Miller, R.E., and Zintel, H.A.   Juvenile polyps of the colon. *Surgery* 69(2):288, 1971.

Holgersen, L.O., Mossberg, S.H., and Miller, R.E.   Colonoscopy for rectal bleeding in childhood. *J. Pediatr. Surg.* 13:83, 1978.

Liebman, W.M.   Fiberoptic endoscopy of the gastrointestinal tract in infants and children: I. Upper endoscopy in 53 children. *Am. J. Gastroenterol.* 68:362, 1977.

Liebman, W.M.   Fiberoptic endoscopy of the gastrointestinal tract in infants and children: II. Fiberoptic colonoscopy and polypectomy in 15 children. *Am. J. Gastroenterol.* 68:452, 1977.

Liebman, W.M., Thaler, M.M., and Bujanover, T.   Endoscopic evaluation of upper gastrointestinal bleeding in the newborn. *Am. J. Gastroenterol.* 69:607, 1978.

Tedesco, F.J.   Upper gastrointestinal endoscopy in the pediatric patient. *Gastroenterology* 70:492, 1976.

CHAPTER 10

OTHER FIBEROPTIC TECHNIQUES

ENTEROSCOPY

The midgut (that is, the jejunum and ileum) has been a no-man's land for endoscopists. The duodenoscope reaches into the fourth portion of the duodenum and the colonoscope can be introduced into the ileocecal valve for examination of the terminal ileum, but all the intestinal territory between remains unexplored.

Some success has been achieved in extending the inspection of the small bowel. The available techniques of small bowel endoscopy are the following:

1. Peroral jejunal endoscopy with a long colonoscope
2. Passive peroral intubation with a prototype long enteroscope
3. Transintestinal catheter guide for
   a. Pulling attached endoscope
   b. Forceps channel monorail passage
4. Intraoperative manipulation after peroral or peranal intubation
5. Intubation of an ileostomy stoma
6. Colonoscopic intubation of the ileocecal valve

Gaisford has employed the 186-cm Olympus colonoscope (CF-LB) for jejunal examination. The proximal half of the jejunum was visualized with this instrument introduced in the usual peroral manner. In Japan, a 10-mm-caliber endoscope 162 cm in length has been similarly employed to study the upper jejunum.

Examination of the ileum has been a more challenging problem. Although the distal 20 to 30 cm of ileum can be intubated colonoscopically in many patients, most of the ileum has remained out of view except on the few occasions when ileoscopy was performed via an ileostomy, or when an endoscope has been manipulated into the small bowel by the operating surgeon during laparotomy.

Small bowel intubation was accomplished by Wolff and Shinya who introduced perorally a long Olympus small intestinal balloon-tipped endoscope, which by passive intubation over hours or days reached the distal ileum much in the way a Miller-Abbott tube will traverse the bowel. Examination of the mucosal surface is made as the instrument is withdrawn, but unfortunately the design of the instrument does not permit biopsy or aspiration for cytology.

Because passive intubation is not dependable, a monorail technique has been employed to bring the endoscope into place in a reasonable and predictable time. This method requires the patient to swallow a small bore catheter with a mercury-weighted tip. When the catheter tip is retrieved in the rectum, the catheter then serves as a transintestinal guide wire for the endoscope, which may be a long bundle colonoscope or a 10-mm-diameter prototype enteroscope with a working length of over 2 meters. The orad end of the catheter is pulled through the forceps channel of the endoscope, which is then advanced over the guide through the entire small intestine under fluoroscopic control. Of course the catheter tip may be merely attached to the end of the endoscope, which would then be pulled into the small intestine by traction of the catheter at the anus.

Under what circumstances is it reasonable to ask a patient to undergo this long and tedious examination of the small intestine? The most obvious situation is one where the site of chronic blood loss has not been identified despite the deployment of the total diagnostic armamentarium, including upper and lower digestive tract endoscopy and selective mesenteric angiography. Bleeding lesions that may be encountered are benign polypoid neoplasms, lymphoma or carcinoma, angiomata, and Meckel's diverticulum. In view of the frustration experienced by surgeons in the search for small bowel lesions at laparotomy, a preoperative (or intraoperative) endoscopic diagnosis may prevent a negative exploration for a small bowel bleeding lesion.

Another indication for enteroscopy is to establish the diagnosis of Crohn's disease of the small bowel. Some patients with suspected regional enteritis have a small bowel series that is not diagnostic, and enteroscopy would provide a visual as well as histologic diagnosis. On occasion, changes in small bowel x-rays are not conclusive, and enteroscopy might provide confirmation of ileitis, lymphoma, lymphoid hyperplasia, or tuberculosis.

It is clear that routinely successful endoscopy of the small bowel is not presently obtainable. However, available instruments will permit extension of the readily visualized portion of the gastrointestinal tract. Much ingenuity in this regard has already been demonstrated, and it is anticipated that advances in instrument design and the use of drugs such as metoclopramide to speed transit time of the enteroscope will make enteroscopy a routine procedure in the future.

CHOLEDOCHOSCOPY

Fortunately, retained bile duct stones are an uncommon occurrence following cholecystectomy and intraoperative cholangiography, but it is by no means a rare event. In the past, intraoperative choledochoscopy never achieved popularity because of the difficulty with instrumentation, but with the recent development of a flexible fiberoptic choledochoscope there has been a resurgent interest in this technique. Indeed, the instrument may also be used for patients in whom common bile duct stones are found postoperatively, by introducing the choledochoscope via the T–tube tract into the common bile duct. Should both the intraoperative and postoperative choledochoscopy be technically impossible or not performed for some reason, choledochoscopy can still be done in certain centers with the prototype thin flexible fiberendoscope passed via the duodenoscope through the papilla of Vater for visualization of the bile ducts. Finally, if retained common bile duct stones have been demonstrated, endoscopic papillotomy can be done for spontaneous passage or extraction.

Instrumentation

The Olympus Model CHF-B3 has a working length of 280 mm with a short rigid proximal section and a flexible longer distal section (see Fig. 10-1). It measures 6.5 mm in diameter, and has an irrigation channel of 2.6 mm. The tip can be bent 100 degrees up and down, and the optical system has an angle view of 65 degrees with depth of field 3 to 50 mm. (The Machida Endoscope Company and Fujinon Optical Company manufacture choledochoscopes of similar design.) The design of the instrument has been modified because some surgeons found the shaft of the instrument too flexible and the entry port of the channel too near the unsterile face mask of the operator. The entry port

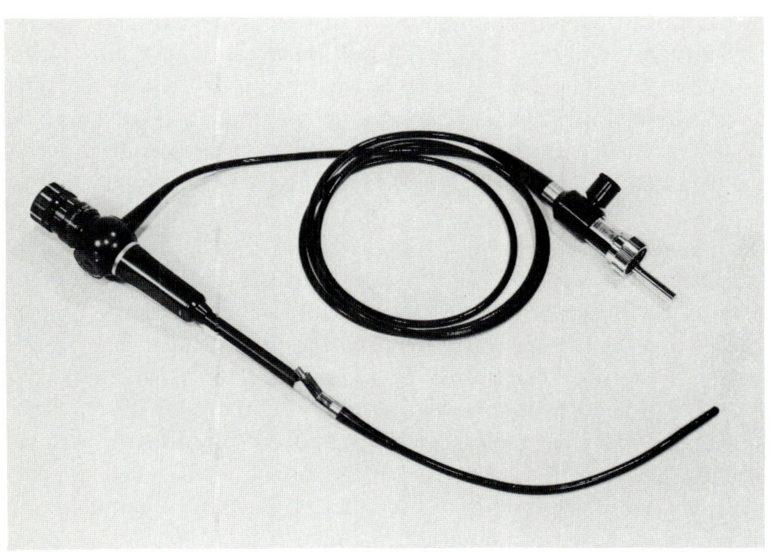

Figure 10-1.   Olympus CHF-B3 choledochoscope.

of the irrigation channel has been relocated to the proximal end of the flexible segment away from the surgeon's face. The fiberoptic instrument must be sterilized by ethylene oxide gas, and this represents its major disadvantage over the older rigid instrument.

Technique of Intraoperative Choledochoscopy

Exploration of the common bile duct is not a failsafe method of assuring complete absence of retained calculi in the biliary tree. When the surgeon palpates the duct or probes in search of stones, he is obviously at a disadvantage with these insensitive manipulations. Cholangiography during surgery presents a difficulty in technique and interpretation of the cholangiogram and, although it is a more satisfactory evaluation of the biliary tree than can be made manually, it is not a foolproof approach. Direct visualization thus offers the best means of clearing the bile ducts of calculi.

Obviously, intraoperative cholangiography will be done only by an experienced surgeon who is familiar with the indications and contraindications for bile duct exploration by any method. If a good preoperative cholangiogram has not been obtained by either ERCP or percutaneous transhepatic cholangiography, then a preliminary operative cholangiogram should be done by passing a fine catheter via the cystic duct into the common bile duct. After the cholecystectomy is completed, the common bile duct is explored as usual; any stones encountered are removed. The choledochoscope is then passed into the common bile duct, and irrigation with normal saline begins. The hepatic ducts are visually examined first, then the instrument is passed into the distal common bile duct which can be studied in almost every case if continuous irrigation is maintained so that the lumen remains open.

With the Olympus CHF-B3 choledochoscope, which allows one-handed manipulation of the controls, stone extraction is possible under direct vision using a balloon catheter or wire basket. Some surgeons believe that when a satisfactory choledochoscopy has been performed, the common bile duct may be closed without a T-tube drain.

Postoperative Choledochoscopy

In patients who have a T tube in place and a postoperative cholangiogram demonstrating retained stones, choledochoscopy may be performed by passing the instrument via the T-tube tract. The T-tube tract, however, must be dilated to a diameter greater than 22 French if the choledochoscope is to be passed into the common bile duct. Since dilation may take as much as 4 to 5 weeks to accomplish, the surgeon might use a large T tube initially in anticipation of a retained stone, both of these procedures being a rather unsatisfactory alternative to successful intraoperative choledochoscopy.

Conclusions

It is evident that if at least 5 percent of patients have retained stones following conventional exploration of the bile ducts, there is a place for a better technique of exploration. Several surgeons have reduced the incidence of retained common bile duct stones to less than 1 percent with intraoperative choledochoscopy. Ashby had a series of 50 patients free of retained stones postoperatively, and he is so confident that a successful choledochoscopy can exclude intraductal stones that he no longer inserts a T-tube drain after choledochoscopic exploration of the bile ducts. If this experience is confirmed by other surgeons, it is likely that intraoperative choledochoscopy will become a routine technique for bile duct exploration.

EXPERIMENTAL ENDOSCOPY

It is noteworthy that the clinical feasibility of the first fiberoptic gastroscope was not tested in an animal. Indeed, after years of clinical application, when fiberoptic endoscopy was determined to be an eminently safe procedure in man, it was extensively used for experimental purposes in animals. The earliest animal endoscopy was probably carried out in the pig for clinical evaluation rather than for experimental purposes, since the pig is peculiarly susceptible to the development of gastric ulcers. Veterinarians performed fiberoptic gastroscopy for the diagnosis of this porcine disease.

Various animals have been used for investigative purposes as well as for designing or learning new endoscopic techniques. Rats have proven to be good gastroscopic subjects, and induced gastric ulceration has been studied in these animals with the use of fiberscopes measuring only a few mm in diameter, and designed primarily for arthroscopy. A similar instrument has been utilized for the purpose of evaluating therapy of chemically-induced rodent colitis, the healing of which can be observed colonoscopically.

The chimpanzee has been studied, after appropriate general anesthesia, with a standard fiberoptic gastroscope. For smaller animals, such as a monkey, rabbit, or rat, a bronchoscope is adaptable for examination of the esophagus and the stomach.

Reports in the literature have described experiences with upper gastrointestinal endoscopy of mammals such as dolphins and killer whales. These procedures have been carried out with rather elaborate preparation and the assistance of veterinarians, primarily for the purpose of determining the best method for removal of foreign bodies from the stomach.

Most of the experimental work performed in recent years has been in anesthetized dogs. In 1970, Goodale et al. described the CO_2 wave laser gastroscope for the control of bleeding gastric erosions induced in dogs. The following year, Sugawa et al., by a transerosal intramural injection of acetic acid, produced acute gastric ulcers observed by serial gastroscopy of the dogs. The healing of the ulcer in a control group was then compared to the healing of the ulcer in dogs receiving systemic histamines, aspirin, steroids, or alcohol. In 1974, Sugawa et al. produced gastric cancer in dogs by the oral administration of a carcinogen (MNNG), and studied the effects of this carcinogen on the healing of experimentally created gastric ulcers (see Fig. 10-2).

The development of endoscopic laser photocoagulation has brought about considerable research in several centers in the United States in the control of standardized experimental gastric bleeding lesions in heparinized dogs. Through a gastrotomy incision, made with the dog under general anesthesia, ulcers are produced by suction biopsy of the mucosa and bleeding is maintained by continuous heparin intravenous infusion. Employing this canine bleeding ulcer model, various laser modalities have been compared to determine effectiveness and safety. The Nd-Yag laser and the argon laser are currently under intensive evaluation in the animal model to determine which is most appropriate for clinical application.

Another approach to the control of upper gastrointestinal bleeding

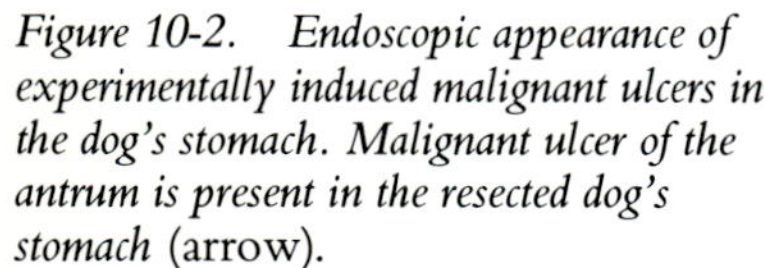

Figure 10-2.   Endoscopic appearance of experimentally induced malignant ulcers in the dog's stomach. Malignant ulcer of the antrum is present in the resected dog's stomach (arrow).

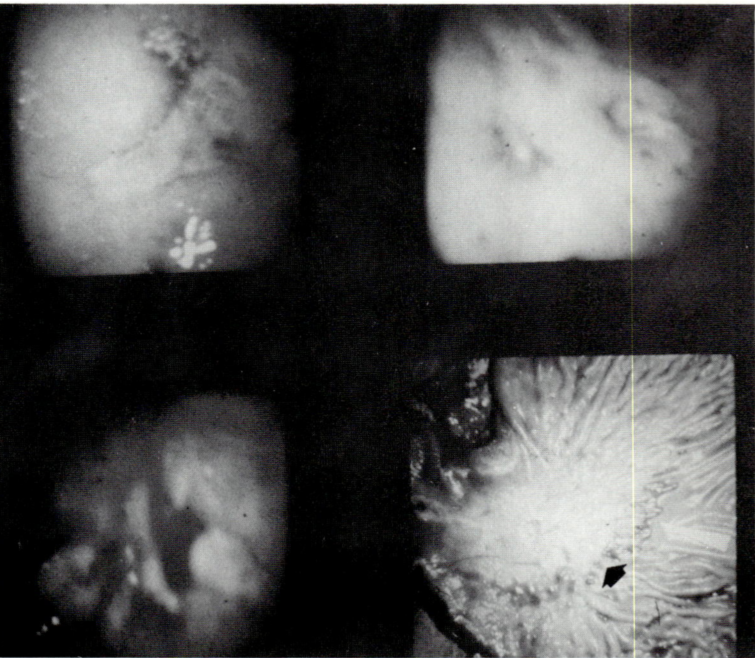

has involved spraying fibrin and cryoprecipitate on the bleeding ulcer of the heparinized canine model. The four-lumen spray tube is passed through the biopsy channel of a standard gastroscope, which is aimed at the bleeding site. This method has been effective in promptly controlling venous bleeding. The canine bleeding ulcer model has also been utilized for the evaluation of electrocoagulation, tissue adhesives, and heater probes. However, it should be noted that not all of these experiments have utilized peroral gastroscopy to test the technique, but rather have merely placed the gastroscope into the stomach through a gastrotomy.

An experiment requiring peroral fiberoptic esophagoscopy was performed in dogs with surgically created esophageal varices, and was designed to demonstrate the effect of the endoscopic injection of sclerosing agents into the varices. The results of this experiment indicated that endoscopic injections of sclerosing agents into esophageal varices can be a safe and reliable technique in the seriously bleeding patient.

It is clear that animal research utilizing fiberoptic endoscopy will play an increasingly important role in the evaluation of new endoscopic instruments, as well as the application of therapeutic modes. Experimental endoscopy permits the performance of techniques that, on the surface, may appear too dangerous to initiate in humans. An apparently unsafe procedure, however, can be modified into one which might prove to be appropriate for clinical trial. The student of fiberoptic endoscopy should make an effort to be familiar with animal investigative work since, in the future, it may be necessary that innovative endoscopic techniques developed in animal models will require physicians who wish to learn the technique to develop their skills by practice in animals.

SELECTED READINGS

Ashby, B.S.   Choledochoscopy. *Clin. Gastroenterol.* 7(3):685, 1978.

Burhenne, H.J.   The technique of biliary duct stone extraction. *Radiology* 113:567, 1974.

Classen, M., et al.   Peroral enteroscopy of the small and large intestine. *Endoscopy* 4:157, 1972.

Deyhle, P., et al.   Endoscopy of the whole small intestine. *Endoscopy* 4:155, 1972.

Goodale, R.L., et al.   Rapid endoscopic control of bleeding gastric erosions by laser radiation. *Arch. Surg.* 101:211, 1970.

Mahood, W.H.   Experimental endoscopy. *Gastrointest. Endosc.* 18(2):83, 1971.

Martin, T.R., Oustad, G.R., and Silvis, S.E.   Endoscopic control of massive upper gastrointestinal bleeding with a tissue adhesive (MBR 4197). *Gastrointest. Endosc.* 24:74, 1977.

Nagasako, K., Yazawa, C., and Takemoto, T.   Biopsy of the terminal ileum. *Gastrointest. Endosc.* 19:7, 1972.

Nora, P.F., et al.   Operative choledochoscopy: Results of a prospective study in several institutions. *Am. J. Surg.* 133:105, 1977.

Protell, R.L., et al.   A reproducible animal model of acute bleeding ulcer . . . The "ulcer maker." *Gastroenterology* 71:961, 1976.

Sugawa, C., et al.   Endoscopic sclerosis of experimental esophageal varices in dogs. *Gastrointest. Endosc.* 24:114, 1978.

Sugawa, C., Lucas, C.E., and Walt, A.J.   Serial endoscopic observation of the effects of histamine, aspirin, steroids and alcohol on standardized gastric ulcers in dogs. *Gastrointest. Endosc.* 18(2):56, 1971.

Sugawa, C., Lucas, C.E., and Walt, A.J.   Serial endoscopic evaluation of experimental gastric cancer. *Gastrointest. Endosc.* 20(3):105, 1974.

Yamakawa, T., Komaki, F.L., and Shikata, J.   Biliary tract endoscopy with an improved choledochofiberscope. *Gastrointest. Endosc.* 24:110, 1978.

INDEX